Carers Handbook Series

Caring for someone with cancer

Toni Battison

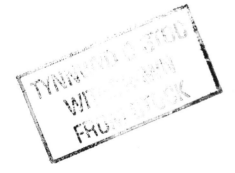

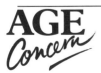

AGE *Concern*

BOOKS

© 2002 Toni Battison
Published by Age Concern England
1268 London Road
London SW16 4ER

First published 2002
Reprinted 2003, 2004

Editor Marion Peat
Production Vinnette Marshall
Designed and typeset by GreenGate Publishing Services, Tonbridge, Kent
Printed in Great Britain by Bell & Bain Ltd, Glasgow

A catalogue record for this book is available from the British Library.
ISBN 0-86242-382-1

Contents

About the author

Toni Battison is a trained nurse who has had considerable practical and teaching experience during her career working with older people and carers, including that of District Nursing Sister, Health Promotion Advisor and Health Lecturer for a Certificate in Health Education course. She is now retired from the NHS and works as a Manager of a charity alongside her freelance health information work. Toni has written many publications promoting good health and is a regular contributor to Radio Cambridgeshire. She is an Associate Member of the Guild of Health Writers.

Toni has always been concerned about the need to support carers and patients to enable them get the best from local and national services as she believes that people obtain great benefit from being able to help themselves. Whilst working for the Cambridge & Huntingdon Health Authority she helped create an information centre for patients and visitors at Addenbrooke's Hospital and, with other carers, started the Telephone Information Line for Carers of Elderly people, in the Cambridge area. She was joint winner of the Ian Nichol Prize for Health Promotion in 1990 and 1992 for these projects.

Toni lives near Cambridge with her husband and mother and has three grown up daughters. Her mother had chemotherapy treatment for stomach cancer at 83 years of age with Toni and her sister sharing the main caring role. She also helped her mother care for her father, after he suffered a stroke, until he died at home. Her time spent as a personal carer has given a different perspective that complements her professional role.

Acknowledgements

The author thanks the many people – carers, colleagues and family members – who have contributed valuable help and advice towards the production of this book. In particular:

Dr P J Wand, Consultant in Palliative Medicine, Medical Director, Marie Curie Centre, Caterham.

A Macmillan Nurse and a carer from the Macmillan Centre, Cambridge.

East Cambridgeshire Older People and Physical Disabilities Team (Social Services).

Staff members of Age Concern England and Scotland for their support and advice throughout the stages of publication, especially Richard Holloway and Vinnette Marshall.

In addition I thank all the national organisations that offer information and support to carers in the broadest sense, whose materials have helped to inform and influence my thinking.

Introduction

Learning that someone close to you has been told he or she has cancer produces many reactions: Is it curable? Will she die? What will happen to her? Will she need treatment and what will it mean? How will we cope? And often carers and relatives are left feeling lost and frightened not knowing where to go for information, advice, help and support. This book attempts to help by providing information to answer some of these questions.

Coping becomes possible when you know what it is you are coping with, and so early chapters explain what cancer is, the symptoms that can lead to the tests to diagnose cancer, the sorts of investigations that may be needed and the various options for treatment. These are described from the perspective of the person facing these tests. The 'natural history' of cancers arising from different parts of the body differ and so the behaviour of the common cancers are outlined with information about the tests that may be needed and treatment that might be offered.

The task of caring falls to many people, both professionals and informal carers, but the greatest part of caring falls to those who are closest to the person involved. The prospect of caring can be daunting. How will you cope with the emotional challenge of being alongside your relative or friend who faces a life-threatening illness, what do you say and will you say the right thing? How will you manage the physical care, especially if you are not very fit yourself? Where can you go for help and what sort of help is available? These are common anxieties and problems and this book will help you find the help you need and explain the roles of all the various agencies (both statutory and voluntary) available. It also will give you practical advice on how to manage to help your relative to be more comfortable and how to help encourage her independence and rehabilitation through treatment and afterwards. Your needs as a carer are considered with suggestions as to how to look after yourself and your own wellbeing.

Many people recover completely after cancer treatment, but some people do not and there is advice as to what happens when cancer progresses and the options for palliative care and further treatment. Looking after someone as they near the end of their life may be stressful and difficult, but it can also be a special and rewarding time for all concerned if the right support is available: this is a period in our lives when time is very precious. Knowledge of what is happening and why, what to expect and how to manage will help to enrich this experience both for you as a carer and for your relative, and it is with this in mind that this book has been written.

Dr P J Wand FRCP, FRCR
Consultant in Palliative Medicine
Medical Director
Marie Curie Centre
Caterham

1 What do you know about cancer?

A diagnosis of cancer invariably triggers strong emotions, leaving everyone involved feeling scared and confused. Initial reactions may vary, but most people express shock and disbelief and often ask the same questions over and over again: 'Why my husband? What did we do wrong? What can we do about this dreadful thing that is happening to us?'

When faced with such a situation you may find it helpful to do something positive, because taking action helps you regain a sense of control. Here, then, is a chance for you, in your role as carer, to begin doing something practical. Gathering information about cancer will provide some answers about what's happening now and what might happen in the future. It's a task that you can undertake, on behalf of yourself and your relative, because it is unlikely that they will feel up to exploring the topic themselves.

This book offers general advice about caring and some basic information about cancer. If you would like to know more about cancer there are many books available that deal with the subject in greater depth. The particular cancer that your relative suffers from may not be mentioned by name in this book but that does not make it less important. The whole topic of 'cancer' is very complex. The text should go a long way towards answering your questions; however, it

1

may also raise uncertainties about other issues that you could explore further by asking the cancer team treating your relative, or by contacting one of the cancer helplines listed on pages 258–274.

Some of the medical terms used in the book are technical. A glossary explaining some less well-known words can be found on pages 253–257.

What is cancer?

Cancer is not a single disease as the name suggests but a general term covering many different types of malignant tumours. There are over two hundred types of cancer, each is distinctive, with its own symptoms and characteristics determined by the sort of cancer it is and where it arises in the body. With all the different cancers around it is no wonder that people are confused about the illness; add to this the tradition of public silence and folklore and you have a recipe for fear.

Cell division

All cancers start in the same way. The information that controls the growth of a normal body cell goes wrong, the message to the cell is altered and from that point onwards that cell grows abnormally. The human body is composed of tissues and organs that are made up of collections of specialised cells, around ten billion in the average person. Most of these are replaced regularly as new cells grow to take the place of those that are worn out. This action happens through a process called **cell division**, directed by a central nucleus in each cell that controls its behaviour. The mechanism for all cell division is the same, although the resulting cell for each organ looks different when examined under a microscope.

Cancer starts when the process of cell division goes wrong; this begins in an individual cell. In fact this abnormal process happens regularly but the body usually recognises very early on that something is wrong and destroys the rogue cell. When a cancer develops the body has failed to recognise that the cells are flawed and has not destroyed the abnormal cells. Gradually, the number of abnormal cells increases and a cluster or lump of cells develops. The time it takes for the lump to be big enough to be noticed depends very much on where in the body it starts to grow; for example, a skin lump will be noticed very quickly but a tumour deep inside the body may remain undetected until it has grown to a size where it causes symptoms. To date, doctors and scientists researching into the reasons for abnormal changes in cell growth do not fully understand how or why it happens.

Benign and malignant tumours

The word tumour means lump and may be used to describe any swelling; it does not mean that the growth is a cancer (a **malignant** tumour). Most lumps or tumours are not cancers (**benign** tumours).

So what is it that decides whether a lump is a benign tumour or is a cancer? This is not always an easy question to answer. Malignant tumours have certain features which make them easier to recognise:

- Cells grow in a disordered fashion – more than are needed to replace dead cells.
- The clumps of cells grow into nearby structures, they invade these structures and grow out of the organ they have arisen from.
- The cells can grow along nerves, and grow into blood vessels and lymphatic vessels.
- Cells can break off the parent tumour and travel across the cavities in the body (for example, the cavity in the tummy where all the abdominal organs lie).
- Cells invade blood and lymphatic vessels so little collections of abnormal cells can travel to different parts of the body.

Benign tumours share none of these characteristics. Although benign tumours can grow very large, they remain in the original organ even though the lump might get quite squashed. Benign tumours do not invade other structures and do not travel to different parts of the body.

In practice, the difference between benign and malignant cells can be very slight, which is why doctors need to do a range of tests to reach a decision.

The only way that a doctor can be sure of the difference between a malignant and a non-malignant tumour is by examining a part of the lump under a microscope, to see the pattern of growth and to look at the cells in fine detail.

Why 'cancer'?

As part of your curiosity about the disease you may wonder how it came to be named. The word originates from Roman times when ancient writers described an incurable, ulcer-like disease that spread into a shape resembling a crab; 'cancer' is the Latin word for crab. Other words you will frequently hear and read are 'tumour' meaning a lump; 'neoplasm' meaning new tissue and 'oncology' which means the study of swellings. An 'oncologist' is a doctor specialising in cancer treatment. Another word 'carcinoma' has entered our language, taken from the writings of Hippocrates, and meaning a malignant growth.

John, a doctor

'I am aware of the enormous effort it takes for some patients to say the word "cancer". I hear the disease talked about much more mysteriously. Common phrases are spoken in hushed tones that leaves no one in any doubt about what is being discussed, but the taboo word "cancer" is rarely mentioned; "the Big C" and "that dreaded disease" are terms that spring to mind.'

What causes cancer?

There are many known facts and a great deal of fiction about what causes cancer – and most people will know a little of both. Most families have experienced cancer near at hand so it's not surprising that people have gathered information along the way, picked up from word of mouth, the television and magazines. Unfortunately, not all information passed around is entirely accurate and the myths that circulate can result in people believing wrongly about the causes and control of the disease. This may cause people to suffer unnecessary guilt and anxiety – about whether or not they caused their own cancer and about how the course of the illness will run. For example, it is commonly supposed that having cancer implies a lingering and painful death, which is not true.

It is true that the number of people diagnosed with cancer is increasing; there are reasons for this that will be explained later. Fortunately, it is also true that treatments are improving continually and many cancers, such as Hodgkin's disease (see page 46), that would have been fatal in the past, can now often be cured.

Understanding the facts

■ Cancer is not one but many different diseases with different causes; for example, chemicals in tobacco smoke cause lung cancer but these do not cause breast cancer.
■ Cancers are caused by substances known as **carcinogens**: materials that are found commonly in the environment to which our bodies are exposed, over a period of time. Two centuries ago a man named Percival Potts linked the development of cancer of the scrotum to chimney sweeps but it was not until the twentieth century that scientists found a carcinogen in soot.
■ Studies by scientists over the years have shown that certain groups of people are more prone to some kinds of cancers than other people; genetics (family history) and environmental issues both play a part in this disease pattern.

5

- Cancer rates differ in countries around the world. By comparing Japanese people with people in the UK it is known that the Japanese death rate for stomach cancer is double that of people in England and Wales, whilst the death rate for breast cancer is very much higher in this country.
- There is sufficient, proven evidence available to accurately pinpoint the cause of some cancers deriving from what people eat, their behaviour, how they live and the relationship with their work; for example, asbestos is a known work-related carcinogen.

Correcting the fiction

Lisa, a doctor

'Unfortunately, people seem to remember the fiction rather than the fact and this can increase their anxiety. If you are unclear, ask the medical team to repeat the information. We would much rather do this than let patients leave with the wrong idea about their cancer.'

- **Myth:** Cancer always means a premature death. **Correction:** No, a diagnosis of cancer does not always mean a death sentence, particularly if the tumour is found at an early stage. Many types of cancer that were incurable 20 years ago are now completely treatable.
- **Myth:** Cancer is caused by injuries such as knocks and bumps. **Correction:** This is definitely not true; however, there is a slight connection in that a painful knock may make the person more aware of the tender area and that leads to them feeling a lump that was already there.
- **Myth:** Cancer is contagious, meaning it can be caught from someone else by touching them or giving them a hug. **Correction:** It is impossible to catch most cancers through everyday contact with another person so don't be afraid to visit friends and relatives in hospital and give them a special hug of comfort.

■ **Myth:** Cancer is hereditary in families. **Correction:** Few types of cancer are hereditary; some rare forms of cancer can be inherited.

■ **Myth:** Cancer is caused by stress. **Correction:** There is no evidence that links the development of cancer to any mental or emotional upset.

■ **Myth:** Women are more at risk of developing cancer than men. **Correction:** Figures show that the risks are similar and the main types of cancer are the same. Men and women die fairly equally from cancers of the stomach, large intestine and pancreas. The difference is found in the cancers linked to specific, gender-related organs, such as the prostate gland in men and ovaries or womb in women.

Risk factors

There are several risk factors that are linked to the chances of developing cancer; some are avoidable, some are controllable, whilst others are pre-determined. Experiments have shown the links to known carcinogens beyond reasonable doubt, so it is a fact that changes in lifestyle can prevent or reduce significantly the risk of developing some cancers. Experts have estimated that the majority of cancers (80 per cent) may be preventable if people take avoiding action (see 'Screening for cancer' on page 14).

Age

Older people are healthier and better cared for than ever before so the balance of the age of the population in the UK is changing. Fewer deaths from other causes has led to an increase in the incidence of cancer, which is predominantly a disease of ageing bodies.

Lisa, a doctor

'Fortunately, the growth rate for most cancers is slower in older people than in the younger age group.'

Family history

Few cancers are inherited in the same way as some other diseases, such as haemophilia or Huntingdon's chorea. However, it is a common observation that certain cancers seem to run in families; for example breast, ovarian and bowel tumours. There is now evidence that certain families do carry genes that make it more likely that family members will develop cancer compared with the general population. (Genes form the 'code' that is carried in each cell in the body, with the instructions for how that individual will be formed and their unique characteristics). So, although the familial tendency to develop cancer may be genetically determined for some cancers, it's also likely that a family shares certain lifestyle behaviour (such as diet or smoking) making them more prone to developing the disease.

Exposure to carcinogens

Long-term contact with certain chemicals, for example coal tar, is well proven as a risk to developing cancer. Since this particular carcinogen was first researched over half a century ago, many other chemicals have been identified that damage cells and trigger cancer. Health and safety measures in most occupations are now excellent so the risks of cancer from exposure to chemical pollutants is very low; however, the effects of past contact with substances such as asbestos may still lie dormant in some people.

For the ordinary person the risk of long-term exposure to most chemical carcinogens is minimal, apart from one serious exception – exposure to cigarette smoke. Tobacco contains thousands of different chemicals, many of which are very toxic. Smoking is the biggest avoidable cause of ill health and premature death in the UK. Over one hundred people die each day of lung cancer, with 81 per cent of these deaths attributable to smoking.

Diet

It has been estimated that up to 35 per cent of cancers may be linked to what we eat, particularly tumours of the digestive tract, the breast and the prostate gland. There is a strong belief held by nutritionists that diets rich in fresh fruit and vegetables help to protect us against these and other cancers. The exact reasons are not fully known; there may be a connection with their high vitamin content but until continuing research brings firmer answers the general message is to eat a selection of fresh produce daily. There is no evidence that vitamin or mineral supplements can bring extra protection, over and above that provided by those found naturally in fresh food. Neither is there any evidence as yet that artificial colourings, flavourings or preservatives are the cause of cancer. Research and testing continues with many dietary products.

The high incidence of breast and bowel cancers in the UK may be connected to the high fat diet that many people consume, rich in animal fats. There may also be a link between obesity and certain cancers: the breast and womb in women and the prostate gland in men. For women this risk escalates after the menopause. Eating more foods high in fibre and starch, and reducing the amount of saturated fats eaten may offer protection against bowel cancer.

Alcohol

The number of people who die from cancers related to alcohol consumption is much lower than those related to smoking but there is a risk which is avoidable. The connection between alcohol and cancer is not straightforward as it seems to depend on a number of contributing factors; for example, the amount of alcohol drunk, whether cigarette smoking is combined with alcohol, and certain dietary factors. Around three per cent of all cancers are thought to be as a result of an excessive intake of alcohol, including cancer of the throat, mouth and oesophagus (gullet).

9

Viruses

In simple terms, it is correct to say that cancer is not infectious; it is not spread around like colds or influenza. However, certain viruses are believed to play a role in the development of *some* cancers. Cancer of the liver (linked to the hepatitis B virus) and cancer of the cervix (associated with the human papilloma virus) are examples of cancers that are related to viruses, although infection with the virus will have taken place long before the cancer develops. Fortunately, these are not very infectious viruses and are only transmitted by very close human contact (usually through sexual intercourse) or through the transfusion of blood or blood products. People infected with the Human Immuno-deficiency Virus (HIV) who develop Acquired Immune Deficiency Syndrome (AIDS) are also more likely to develop some forms of cancer, such as Kaposi's sarcoma and lymphomas (see 'Glossary' on pages 253–257). Research into cancers related to viruses continues; however, in the majority of cancers there is no evidence at present that viruses are involved.

Hormones

Hormones, or 'chemical messengers', are substances made and secreted by glands in the body to trigger other organs into action. Hormone therapy has been prescribed for many years to alter body functions; the role of hormones is an integral part of virtually all body functions, an example is in male and female sexual development. The effects of hormones produced within the body can be modified; taking the contraceptive pill to prevent ovulation is one example of hormone interference. Certain cancers are influenced by hormones, for example prostate cancer. Androgens, male sex hormones, promote the growth of prostate cancer and if these hormones are removed by castration then the cancer will usually respond by stopping growing and shrinking. Another example is breast cancer, where the age at which a woman started having her periods, when she had her babies and whether or not she breast fed them are thought to have some influence on whether or not she will develop breast cancer.

The media is quick to report any controversy over the links between hormone intervention and the incidence of cancer and it's possible that there is a connection. It is now thought that the long-term use of contraceptive pills may be associated with a very tiny increased risk of breast cancer. Much research is being done all over the world into the connection with hormone treatments such as HRT (hormone replacement therapy) but any risks that might be associated with this are likely to be very small compared with the known benefits.

What are the risks of getting cancer?

Fact box

- Over 250,000 people develop cancer annually in the UK.
- 65 per cent of new cancers occur in people aged 65 plus.
- Lung cancer is the single most common cancer (1 in 5 new cases) affecting both men and women in the UK (16 per cent).
- Lung cancer is the single most common cancer affecting males only in the UK (21 per cent).
- Breast cancer is the single most common cancer affecting females only in the UK (27 per cent).
- The risk rate for an individual person developing any cancer in their lifetime is estimated at 1 in 3 now (rising to 1 in 2) because of the influence of an ageing population.

Source: Cancer Research Campaign factsheet 1.1 (1995 figures)

When health professionals talk about cancer they often mention the good news first, followed by the not-so-good news. The good news is that many cancers are preventable, ie the risk rate of developing the disease can be reduced enormously by following a few straightforward rules. The less favourable news is that it is impossible to maintain control over every aspect of your lifestyle. The statistics show that currently about one in three of us will get cancer and about one in four of us will die from cancer. It is predicted that this will increase in the 21st century and that about 1 in 2 people in westernised societies will develop some form of cancer. The main reason for this rise is that despite greater knowledge about cancer and what causes it, cancer remains primarily a disease of older age and the population is getting older.

How do doctors know that a patient has cancer?

All cancers start as a tiny abnormal cell that eventually grows into a lump big enough to be detected. However, this little lump may not produce any symptoms at all or only very vague symptoms and in the early stages of the illness you and your relative may not have suspected anything serious, let alone cancer. However, at some point the symptoms became sufficiently troublesome to lead most people to seek advice.

Although each particular cancer is different, many share similar signs and symptoms. When a person consults with their GP, the doctor will be looking out for certain symptoms that make up an 'early warning' checklist. Depending on the information that the patient gives, the doctor may ask in-depth questions about any of the following:

- persistent coughing and hoarseness;
- blood passed in urine, stools or present in mucus or discharge;
- changes in bowel habits;
- bleeding between periods or after intercourse or after the menopause;
- unusual lumps: in the breast, testicles, neck and any other glands;
- unexplained tiredness, loss of weight, indigestion;
- persistent pain.

On their own, none of the symptoms on this list indicate cancer and each could be caused by another problem. The doctor will send a person for further investigations when he is satisfied that several warning symptoms are present and that they are persistent. The government has issued guidelines to GPs about which symptoms indicate a need for urgent investigation (see below). If your relative has symptoms that suggest they fall within these guidelines then an appointment to be seen by a specialist will be offered within a given time period of being referred by their GP. The NHS Plan launched in July 2000 states that all people with a suspected cancer will be offered an urgent outpatient appointment within a maximum of two weeks.

Government guidelines

In autumn 2000 the Secretary of State for Health launched a comprehensive cancer plan – *A plan for investment. A plan for reform* – that set out the future of NHS cancer services. The action plan outlined a number of measures that included the reduction of waiting times for the treatment of cancer patients; the development of a new National Cancer Research Institute (NCRI); and investment into palliative care and cancer hospices.

One of the main features of the plan was the introduction of target times for the treatment of urgently referred cancers, to be phased in over a period up to 2005.

- A maximum one month wait, from urgent GP referral to treatment, guaranteed for children's and testicular cancers and acute leukaemia by 2001.
- A maximum one month wait, from diagnosis to treatment, for breast cancer by 2002.
- A maximum one month wait, from diagnosis to treatment, for all cancers by 2005.

By this date the maximum one-month wait from diagnosis to commencement of treatment for all types of cancer will be well established. For some cancers this time guarantee is already in practice.

Screening for cancer

Health promotion campaigns inform the public about how to lead healthier lives and protect ourselves against disease. Health screening has been available for many years with some programmes, such as those for breast and cervical screening, demonstrating excellent results. It may seem strange, therefore, that national screening programmes are not set up for other cancers. This question has been debated often; however, screening can only have real benefits if tests:

■ can detect a cancer at an early stage, before it would have presented with symptoms **and** that treatment at this early stage is known to be more effective and to save lives compared with treatment at the time that symptoms develop;
■ are able to detect a high proportion of the early developing cancers;
■ are specific and do not give 'false positives', leading to a great deal of anxiety;
■ are safe, cheap and the results easy to interpret.

At present the UK national screening programmes are directed towards breast and cervical screening.

Cervical screening

A smear test is available free of charge under the NHS to all sexually active women under the age of 65 years, every three to five years, or more frequently depending on the recommendation of the doctor. It is designed to detect pre-cancerous cells in the neck of the womb which can be treated before they become malignant; occasionally the test detects cancer cells and if this happens treatment can be started at a time before the patient has had any symptoms.

Breast screening

A free mammogram (see page 56) is available to all women in the UK under the NHS breast screening programme. The check is cur-

14

rently offered three-yearly (to most women) between the ages of 50 to 64, at specialist centres – often mobile units that tour the area. This will be extended to include women up to age 70, phased in over a three-year period until 2004.

Self-examination for breast cancer

In between x-ray screening, women are advised to do regular self-checks at home at different times of the month. Advice about how to observe and feel the nature of each breast is available at a surgery. It is vital that any irregularities are shown to a GP or breast care nurse. The warning signs to look out for are:

- a painless hard lump in the breast or in the armpit;
- weeping or bleeding from the nipple;
- puckering of the skin or drawing in of the nipple;
- broken areas of skin on the surface of the breast.

Colon cancer

Although cancer of the bowel is one of the commoner cancers, there are no absolutely reliable techniques to enable very early detection. The cancer, which starts in the wall of the colon, must grow to a certain size before blood can be detected in the stools. Chemical substances are available that can detect minute traces of blood on toilet paper; however, there is usually a non-malignant reason for blood in the faeces. Self-help observations include being aware of a few related symptoms:

- visible blood in the stools;
- changes in bowel habits including constipation and diarrhoea; leaking of faecal matter; frequent sensation of needing to empty the bowels and painful anal spasms;
- abdominal pain which is general or more marked in the left lower area;
- feelings of distension and discomfort if the tumour is restricting bowel movement causing a build up of wind and faeces;
- unexplained loss of weight, anaemia and feeling generally unwell.

Prostate cancer

Routine screening is not offered in the UK although a national pro-gramme is available in America based on a blood test. This test is not very specific giving the risk of false positive and false negative results, which is why the test has not been adopted for routine screen-ing in this country. All men need to be aware of early symptoms:

- passing water more often than usual, especially at night;
- a reduction in the flow and force of the urine stream;
- difficulty in starting and stopping the flow with (rarely) a com-plete inability to start;
- blood and pain on passing urine.

These symptoms are not specific for prostate cancer but are indi-cations for your relative to consult their GP.

Testicular cancer

Men should be encouraged to take responsibility for making regu-lar checks as part of a 'body familiar' process, although it is common for partners to undertake this task on their behalf. The best time to do this is after a bath or shower when the scrotum feels relaxed. Hold the scrotum in one hand to check weight and size then feel each testicle in turn with thumb and fingers. Finally, look at the genital area standing in front of a full length mirror, in a good light. Warning signs and symptoms to look out for are:

- lumps and irregularities in shape;
- change in size, shape and density;
- any discharge from the penis.

Skin cancer

The amount of exposure to the sun and the extent of pigmentation (colouring) of the skin are the most important factors affecting the development of skin cancers. The level of protection the body pro-vides is dependent on production of a substance called melanin. Fair skinned people are more at risk because they produce melanin much more slowly than darker skinned people. Skin cancer is very uncommon in Asian, black and olive skinned people because they produce high levels of pigment. Most cases of skin cancer are found in older people after years of exposure to strong sunlight.

The most crucial factor is exposure to strong sunlight. There are a few simple rules to follow that govern the time and intensity of exposure to the sun. Leaflets are available from GP surgeries giving clear guidelines about how to sunbathe safely. Most skin cancers are completely curable if they are detected and treated early. Fortunately, much of surface skin can be viewed fairly effortlessly; the signs to look for are:

■ areas of broken skin that do not heal up, that itch and bleed, particularly on the head and neck;

■ any changes in moles, such as increased growth, changes in shape, patchy appearance with dark and light areas, itching and bleeding.

Diagnostic tests and treatments for cancer

After being told they have cancer, people tend to focus on the immediate future, asking first and foremost about the types of treatment and the possibility that the doctors have made a mistake. The next chapter looks in greater depth at the methods used to confirm the presence of cancer and the main forms of treatment. A brief description is given below of the range of tests and treatments that are used. The methods chosen by the cancer team depend very much on the type of cancer that is suspected, where it lies in the body, how long it has been developing and which treatments are most effective.

■ **Tests:** GPs, surgeons and cancer specialists start by asking the patients to tell the 'story' of their illness, past illnesses and details about their work and lifestyle, and by carrying out a physical examination, to get an early 'picture'. This is followed by a range of tests to make a diagnosis and establish the extent and type of the cancer, if this is suspected. The tests may include blood tests, x-rays which may be simple x-rays or more complicated investigations and, wherever possible, a biopsy.

17

This last test, which involves removing a part of the tumour so that it can be examined under a microscope, is needed to confirm the diagnosis of cancer.

■ **Treatments:** a number of options are available for the specialist to choose depending on the type of cancer that is present, how far it has developed and what is already known to be the most effective combination of therapies. The main choices include surgery, chemotherapy, radiotherapy, hormonal treatment and immuno-therapy. Whether or not the cancer has spread to other parts of the body needs to be checked as this makes a difference to the type of treatment that will be offered.

Types of cancer

All cancers are named by doctors according to the type of cell and the organ from which they developed. Generally the name will give a guide to the sort of cancer it is and where it came from. The following list explains some of the terms that are used.

■ **Carcinoma:** implies that the cancer has arisen in the tissues that are derived from cells that, in the developing embryo, formed the outside skin or the developing gut. These embryonic structures develop into many structures in the adult, including: skin, and areas such as the breast that develop from the skin; the lining of the mouth, throat, lungs, stomach and intestines; glands that make secretions, salivary glands, pancreas and prostate. Carcinomas are by far the commonest types of cancer, and so the term is often used rather loosely to cover all cancers.

■ **Sarcoma:** indicates that the tumour has derived from the 'middle' layer of the embryo which develops into muscles, bones, fibrous tissue and fat.

■ **Lymphoma:** tumours that arise in lymphoid tissue in the body, found in lymph glands, the spleen and the bone marrow, where the blood cells are formed. If the malignant process involves the blood-forming tissues in the bone marrow then leukaemia develops.

The main cancers

John, a doctor

'Fortunately, it isn't necessary for you to remember long, medical words to understand about cancer – but you will hear doctors and nurses using them as they discuss cases with each other. It is quite all right for you and your relative to talk to the doctor about the illness in more everyday language using words that are familiar, for example cancer of the stomach.'

Lisa, a doctor

'The most important information that you need to understand is about the way the cancer is expected to behave and the possible outcome. Prognosis (the word used when forecasting what is likely to happen) depends on a number of factors including the type of cancer that has been diagnosed, how fast that type usually grows, the size of the tumour and whether or not it has spread at the time of diagnosis. If clinical words are used that you or your relative don't understand and you would like a clearer description, do ask a member of the medical team to explain – we won't mind.'

The cancers described in the following section have been included because they are the most common cancers that affect people in the UK. They are grouped under body systems or cancer types as a convenient way of description, starting at the top of each system and working down, where appropriate. Not all body parts are mentioned and the order in which they appear has no bearing on their severity, cause, treatments and chances of recovery. There is no need to read about each cancer – you may wish to move directly to the section that explains your relative's illness in more detail. Some of the medical terms are not commonly known; a glossary explaining many of these special words can be found on pages 253–257.

Respiratory system

Lungs

When theories are put forward about what causes cancer the one example that is irrefutable is the trigger for lung cancer. Most people are aware of the connection between cigarette smoke and the grave risk of developing cancer; other carcinogens such as asbestos contribute to a lesser degree. Until the twentieth century lung cancer was a fairly rare disease in the UK but this pattern changed very significantly after the notable increase in cigarette smoking by men in the 1930s and 1940s. The incidence of lung cancer catapulted into medical awareness in the years after the last war, reflecting the earlier period when men smoked in large numbers. The figures for female lung cancer lag a little behind those of their male peers because women did not start smoking in earnest until during and after the Second World War.

Overall, lung cancer accounts for about one-quarter of all cancer deaths. The evidence over the years suggests that the risk of developing lung cancer is linked to the type and quantity of tobacco smoked and for how long; for example, low tar and filtered cigarettes may reduce the risk whilst a high tar content increases the risk. Cigarette smoking creates a higher risk than pipe or cigar smoking and passive smoking (inhaling the smoke from the tobacco of another person) carries a smaller risk. Other tissue along the pathway of the smoke (throat and bronchial tubes) is also susceptible to damage. For tips on how to give up smoking, see page 118.

Lung cancer falls into several common types affecting the airways, the mucus-producing cells and the lymph gland tissue.

Rarer types do occur, such as the cancer triggered by asbestos.

The signs and symptoms of lung cancer may be picked up at a routine medical examination, or usually as a result of a chest x-ray. The first indications that patients observe are a persistent cough that may be associated with specks of blood in the sputum (phlegm or mucus); shortness of breath; a general feeling of being unwell; weight loss and pain in the chest. However, cancer in the lung often shows no symptoms at the stage where it is most readily treatable, and may not cause problems until it has spread elsewhere in the body.

Investigations start with a chest x-ray which may show a 'shadow' if cancer is present and will lead to further investigations. The sputum may be examined for abnormal cells but usually a bronchoscopy will be carried out to take a biopsy and confirm the diagnosis. Other tests, including a computed tomography (CT) scan, will be performed to determine the extent of the cancer, and other scans may be arranged if it seems likely that the cancer has spread beyond the lungs.

Treatment choices depend largely on the extent to which the cancer has spread and the type of cancer present. Surgery and chemotherapy, followed by radiotherapy are common. If the cancer is too extensive for surgery and the person has no symptoms, then treatment may be held in 'reserve' until symptoms are present.

The outlook for lung cancer patients is improving and a small minority of people are cured or live for several years after treatment. The careful selection of treatment helps to control the symptoms and prolong the lifetime of many patients.

Digestive system

Oesophagus

The incidence of cancer of the oesophagus (gullet) is lower in western countries than some eastern countries, and there is evidence suggesting that environmental factors play a part; poor nutrition and heavy alcohol and cigarette consumption. The cancer first shows as difficulty in swallowing, together with indigestion (heartburn), weight loss and a discomfort in the central chest area. Vomiting may occur not connected with eating and the vomit often contains blood.

These symptoms suggest partial obstruction in the oesophagus and indicate the need for investigation either by endoscopy (looking down the oesophagus with a special instrument) or with an x-ray examination (the patient swallows a barium-containing drink to outline the inside of the gullet). If the oesophagus appears to be obstructed by a tumour shape an endoscopy can be performed to enable the doctor to view the walls of the oesophagus and remove a piece of tissue for biopsy. To prevent any discomfort, endoscopy is carried out whilst the person is sedated but still conscious and able to respond to instructions. A local anaesthetic spray is used to numb the throat area.

Treatment is aimed at removing the tumour through a surgical operation. After surgery the patient may have to adjust their eating habits to eat smaller meals more often and to experiment with softer food if indigestion is a problem. If the tumour has extended beyond the oesophagus (making surgery difficult) either radiotherapy or chemotherapy may be used. One approach is to use chemotherapy in an attempt to shrink the tumour sufficiently to consider surgery.

If the cancer is extensive, chemotherapy alone often helps to improve any symptoms. Other palliative treatments can be offered to help those people who continue to experience difficulty swallowing; for example, the oesophagus can be dilated or a tube can be placed in the oesophagus so that soft food and liquids pass down smoothly. A dietitian will be able to advise the patient and their relatives about sensible eating with this condition.

The forecast is good if the cancer is removed completely and the long-term outlook is much more favourable for people who have had combination therapy.

Stomach

The good news about stomach cancer is that it appears to be declining in western countries; this is a welcome trend but it still remains high on the list of common cancers, affecting males in far greater numbers than females. Like many cancers it is more prevalent in older people and is strongly linked to environmental causes. Some studies being undertaken are investigating food storage methods as the lower incidence in western countries may be due to better food preservation; less smoked or salted foods are eaten in the west than in eastern countries or South America where the incidence is higher. However, this theory is not yet proven and other factors may have a protective action; for example, a diet rich in fresh fruit and vegetables.

Stomach cancer is associated with a number of symptoms that should trigger investigation. Namely, indigestion and a bloated feeling after eating with possible nausea and wind; loss of appetite, weight loss and vomiting (which may be bloodstained) occur at a later stage of the disease; blood may also be noticeable or detectable in the stools. These symptoms are non-specific and occur in other conditions so, whilst they may not be caused by a malignant disease, they should never be ignored or blamed on mere indigestion. Unfortunately, these rather vague symptoms mean that cancers have often developed to a well-advanced stage before treatment commences.

Investigations may start with a barium meal or an endoscopy. The endoscope enables the operator to view the stomach and remove a small sliver of tissue for laboratory examination. This test does not require a general anaesthetic but the patient can be sedated if they choose. If cancer is present further investigations will be carried out, including scans or ultrasound to give an indication of the size and extent of the cancer.

Treatment options will focus on surgery first, as removal of the tumour is important. A partial gastrectomy (removal of part of the stomach) and removal of the lymph glands will be performed, or a total gastrectomy may be carried out. After such operations, help will be available from a dietitian as it takes a while to adjust to radical new eating habits. Chemotherapy is almost always given after surgery and in some cases it is given prior to the operation to reduce the size of the tumour. If surgery is not recommended because of frailty of the patient or spreading of the disease, chemotherapy is helpful in shrinking and controlling the cancer. Radiotherapy is rarely used to treat stomach cancer because of the risk to adjacent organs.

The outlook and prospects for cure are good if the cancer is found and treated early. The chances of long-term survival are less positive for many patients because of the delay in diagnosis; however, life may be prolonged for years. Palliative treatment will ensure that patients whose cancer cannot be cured are offered excellent care and control of symptoms.

Liver

Most people know of someone who has had cancer that involves the liver because it is one of the commonest organs where secondary tumours develop, but it is rarely the site of primary tumours in western societies (although not in Africa and Asia).

Primary cancers grow in two main places in the liver; in the liver cells and the ducts of the liver. Liver cancer tends to develop in middle-age and beyond and is twice as likely to occur in males as females. The cancer may be linked to cirrhosis, a form of liver damage caused by a long history of heavy alcohol drinking or can result from an infection (hepatitis B).

The symptoms arising from cancer involving the liver are a sensation of discomfort and swelling in the upper abdomen often combined with a general feeling of being unwell. If the bile ducts are affected they may become blocked thus preventing bile from passing into the intestines. This causes a rise in the level of bile pigments in the blood causing the person to become jaundiced with marked yellowing of the skin and eyeballs. Other signs of this type of jaundice include itchy skin, dark coloured urine and pale stools. Finally, there may be a build up of fluid within the abdominal cavity, called ascites.

Tests start with a physical examination to enable the doctor to feel the size of the liver. The presence of an enlarged and tender liver will lead them to arrange further tests, such as an ultrasound or a CT scan, to check for further evidence of liver involvement. If the specialist suspects a primary cancer the next steps will be a blood test and a biopsy. If the person is already known to have a primary tumour elsewhere in the body it is usually not necessary to carry out a biopsy.

Treatment of primary liver cancer depends very much on the size of the tumour and to what extent liver function is affected. It is possible to remove a considerable part of the liver (individual lobes) without too much adverse effect on function as the liver is able to repair itself well. Unfortunately, for many patients the cancer is widespread throughout the liver at diagnosis and is too far advanced for safe surgical removal to be possible. Likewise, surgical removal of liver lobes is rarely an option for secondary growths (called metastases) unless these are detected at a very early stage and screening shows that there are no secondary tumours present in other organs.

Chemotherapy can be used to reduce the size of the tumour for a primary cancer. Treatment by chemotherapy for a secondary cancer will be as effective as it was at the primary site. Specialists are currently researching the effectiveness of introducing chemotherapy drugs directly to the liver site by injecting into the artery that feeds blood to the liver. This treatment enables larger doses to be delivered to the liver than would otherwise be possible through the other routes, with fewer side effects. Radiotherapy is rarely used as the liver is very sensitive to radiation; the risk of causing damage to the remaining healthy tissue would be too high. Other newer treatments include injections of alcohol and laser beams to attempt to destroy small secondary tumours.

Liver cancer is difficult to treat whether it is primary or secondary. The main aim of treatments is to control the growth rate of the cancer, relieve the symptoms and give the person as good a quality of life as is possible. A few fortunate people are successfully cured.

Pancreas

Unfortunately, this cancer remains very common, especially in older people. The symptoms for pancreatic cancer are frequently non-specific to start with: poor appetite and weight loss are probably the first indicators, with pain in the upper abdomen and back. If the cancer is growing in the section of pancreas where the bile duct enters, early obstruction may prevent bile passing from the gall bladder to the intestine. The build-up of bile pigments seeps into the bloodstream leading to jaundice. The signs for this condition are very obvious – yellowing of the skin and eyeballs and darker urine whilst the faeces become pale. Jaundice is a symptom that needs investigation, although it does not always mean cancer; there are many conditions causing jaundice.

Investigation starts with a physical examination where the doctor will gently feel the abdominal area for any obvious lumps. The next step is a barium meal x-ray to rule out other possible causes of the symptoms. Additional tests include CT and ultrasound scans to show the extent of the cancer. A biopsy will be carried out to confirm the diagnosis, if possible. This can be done by needle insertion using a local anaesthetic.

Surgery is undertaken if the cancer is not too large and the patient is young and fit. It is possible to remove the whole of the pancreas after which the patient will have to take replacement pancreatic enzymes and insulin for the remainder of their life; however, by the time the diagnosis is made the cancer has often spread to adjoining organs making surgery impossible. Various palliative surgical procedures can be done to ease the situation if the tumour is causing obstruction; for example, to drain or bypass the bile duct. Chemotherapy is increasingly used with good results and hormone therapy and radiotherapy are sometimes used.

If it is not possible to remove the cancer completely, the tumour will be controlled as much as possible and this palliative care includes good pain relief.

Bowel

Bowel cancer, arising from the large bowel (colon and rectum) is very common; it is the second most frequently found cancer in men and the third commonest in women. The chances of getting this type of cancer rise with age. Cancer of the small bowel (duodenum jejunum and ileum) is very rare. Worldwide, the figures for large bowel cancer vary considerably country by country; the numbers of people diagnosed in western countries is similar but global statistics show much lower rates in African and Asian countries. Cancer specialists believe that this type of cancer is closely linked to the lifestyle of people in these wealthier regions with diet playing a major role in causing the disease. Diets in westernised countries tend to be rich in animal meats, fats and alcohol and low in fruit and vegetables, whereas the diets of peoples in less affluent areas of the world are more likely to be rich in fibre and low in animal products.

As well as dietary factors, family history also has a bearing on the chances of developing a cancer of the colon as evidence shows the risks are increased if other family members have been affected, particularly if they developed the cancer at a younger age. The risk is also slightly greater for people who suffer from inflammatory diseases of the bowel, such as Irritable Bowel Syndrome. However, these factors only play a small part towards developing the cancer.

The prognosis for these cancers is very good if they are detected at an early stage when signs and symptoms first appear. The most common signs of the cancer, blood in the stools and altered bowel habits, usually have a simple cause so immediate investigations are vital to rule out a malignant tumour. The investigation of these symptoms starts with examination of the rectum by the doctor, followed by tests to enable the specialist to check the whole bowel and remove a small piece of tissue for biopsy. These special tests may include a sigmoidoscopy (using a rigid instrument to examine the rectum and lower part of the sigmoid colon), or colonoscopy (using a flexible instrument that can examine the whole large bowel). The large bowel can also be examined by x-rays, following a barium enema (see page 56). In order for these investigations to be as thorough as possible, it is necessary to clear out any faecal matter from the bowel and your relative will be given instructions and laxatives to empty the bowel.

Treatment is primarily by surgery with the aim being to remove the section of bowel containing the tumour, together with the surrounding lymph glands, and to join the ends of the bowel back together. Sometimes this is not possible and it may be necessary to perform a colostomy, in which the end of the bowel that is connected to the small bowel is brought out onto the surface of the abdomen. The opening (called a stoma) then empties into a special bag stuck onto the abdominal skin (for management of a stoma, see page 96). The provision of a colostomy may be a temporary or permanent measure depending on several factors, including the extent of the cancer and the surgery that has been carried out. Fortunately, improvements in surgical techniques have now made the fixture of a permanent colostomy much rarer.

Surgery may be combined with radiotherapy or chemotherapy to help reduce the risk of secondary growths occurring. If the cancer does return after the initial treatment then it is nearly always possible to have further treatment with chemotherapy and possibly radiotherapy and, depending on the site of the recurrent disease, further surgery may be performed.

The outlook and life expectancy is very good for those people who are fortunate enough to be first diagnosed when the cancer is at an early stage. For example, if the tumour is detected whilst still within the wall of the bowel the cure rate is about 80 per cent; this falls to around 70 per cent if the cancer has moved beyond the bowel wall but lymph tissue is not yet involved, dropping to between 30 to 50 per cent if lymph glands are involved. Research and advancements in treatment continue and the importance of overcoming fear and embarrassment about seeking early advice should never be overlooked.

Reproductive system – female

Breast

Cancer of the breast is the most common cancer affecting women in the UK. Current figures show that about 1 in 12 women are at risk of developing the disease, so most people know someone who has been affected; its high incidence rate and association with femininity also makes it one of the most feared cancers. There are four main factors that contribute to the risk rate for contracting the disease: the risk increases significantly with age; there is a well established link between hormone levels (mainly oestrogen); family history plays a part with the risk increasing according to the closeness of an affected relative (a mother or sister); and there is a suspected relationship to diet, although there is no hard evidence as yet. An additional, minor factor is the possible connection between breast cancer and a history of repeated mastitis and benign breast cysts. There is no *known* link to accidental damage to the breast.

The female hormone *oestrogen* seems to be a key factor, as women who start their monthly periods (menstruation) early and/or finish late; those that have their first child later in life or those that are childless are more susceptible because of the longer time span that the hormone is in their system. Scientific studies have caused scares in the past by linking the risk rate to use of contraceptive pills containing higher levels of oestrogen; likewise, a small risk is associated with use of hormone replacement therapy during the menopause although it is felt that the benefits outweigh the risks. There is also a belief that a diet high in meat and milk products may help to raise blood levels of oestrogen.

The first detection of breast cancer can be made in several ways, either by the woman (or her partner) feeling a lump, by manual examination at a routine health check or through the mammography breast screening service. No lump should ever be ignored and the good news is that most breast lumps are not cancerous. Lumps are investigated by several methods: mammogram, biopsies (needle and minor surgery), removal of fluid by needle and scans. The course of treatment is decided according to the size and spread of the tumour, whether the lymph glands in the armpit are involved and if there is evidence of spread to other sites in the body. Treatment includes various different surgical approaches to remove the breast lump (lumpectomy, mastectomy and sampling of the lymph nodes in the armpit), and the choice for each woman is decided depending on the stage of the disease and what her preferences are. Most women are offered additional treatment following their surgery. Radiotherapy is offered to women who are treated with 'lumpectomy', and many are treated with a hormone therapy such as Tamoxifen, or chemotherapy, or both. Some older, more frail, women may have breast cancer that is very sensitive to hormone therapy and their tumour may regress with Tamoxifen alone. Breast reconstruction (see page 102) may be considered to restore the shape of the breast.

Treatment for breast cancer that relapses is often very effective for many years and may involve further hormone treatments, further chemotherapy or radiotherapy. The outlook for breast cancer is improving all the time, and the prognosis improves, the earlier the lump is found and treated.

Male breast cancer is rare, but not beyond risk. About two hundred cases a year are diagnosed in the UK, usually in older men, so they should be aware of the signs and symptoms for themselves as well as their partners. Treatments and prognosis rates are similar to those of women.

Cervix

This cancer is now much less common than a few decades ago thanks to the widespread uptake of cervical screening. Early detection of cells still in a pre-cancerous state means that preventative action can be taken before full-blown cancer develops. Women who have been identified in this way are monitored very carefully for many years to ensure that the condition does not regress. Women who have had a hysterectomy no longer need to be tested.

Cancer of the cervix (the neck of the womb) has been linked to several contributing factors. The relationship with sexual activity is notable: the age at which a woman became sexually active and the greater the number of her partners (and her partners' partners), the higher her personal risk becomes. The obvious conclusion is that some component connected with sexual intercourse is partially responsible for triggering the cancer; people who have habitually used barrier methods of contraception (rubber condoms or vaginal caps) seem to be less at risk. Research over the years has looked at the effects of viruses, the contraceptive pill and cigarette smoking.

All probably play a part; for example, women who take the pill rarely use an additional barrier method so it is this factor (rather than the direct effect of the pill) that is meaningful. There are also other unknown factors, so no woman who develops cervical cancer should ever feel badly about her previous lifestyle or blame her partner. The number of women who do not develop cancer, but share a similar history, make the 'guilt' element quite unnecessary.

For women whose cancer is not picked up by a smear test, the warning signs of a possible cancer are bleeding between periods or after intercourse (especially in older women) and a vaginal discharge. Pain is not a symptom of early cancer. All of these symptoms are also indicative of a common, benign condition called cervical erosion, where a small non-malignant ulcer is present on the neck of the womb. It is wise to check out abnormal symptoms however minor they may feel.

Investigation starts with a physical examination of the cervix using an instrument called a speculum. This gently stretches the vaginal channel to enable the doctor to see the cervix and take a small scraping of surface tissue and mucus to send for laboratory testing. The procedure causes little discomfort. The next stage depends on the result of the smear test. Sometimes there are very minor abnormalities present and the patient will be asked to have a repeat test after a period of time to check that these changes have not persisted. If the cells are seen to be abnormal a further test called a colposcopy will be arranged. This is very similar to the examination with the speculum but the instrument used has a magnifying lens allowing more detailed examination. A solution is painted on to the cervix to help identify any abnormal areas so that the doctor can take a small piece of tissue for biopsy. A colposcopy can be done on an outpatient basis but if the cervical area is not easily accessible (it is quite normal for some women to be shaped differently to others) the operation will be done under a general anaesthetic. The surgeon removes a small piece of tissue for examination and depending on the results of this, other tests may be arranged to find out the extent of the disease.

Pre-cancerous cells in the cervix are treated by several different methods: cryotherapy (freezing the cells); diathermy (burning the cells); laser therapy (using light-beams to destroy cells) or cone biopsy (surgical removal of the tissue). All of these methods give excellent results. More advanced cancer is most often treated by surgery, usually a hysterectomy (removing the uterus and lymph nodes), and this may be combined with radiotherapy. Decisions about surgery would always take into account the extent of the disease, the age of the woman and whether or not she wishes to have children. Treatment may be solely by radiotherapy, or by radiotherapy combined with chemotherapy.

Prognosis is very good if the cancer is detected at an early stage with the other treatments providing a good outlook after later diagnosis.

Uterus

Cancer of the body of the uterus (womb) is one of the female cancers that is easily detectable. The cancer mainly affects older women (aged 50 and over). As the majority are past the menopause, the development of bleeding from the vagina will almost certainly ring instant alarm bells. Good media coverage of female health problems means that the majority of women are aware that they should seek advice urgently if bleeding occurs. For younger women the signs of vaginal bleeding between periods should trigger the same investigative action. Pain may be felt in the later stages of the disease if it remains untreated.

The cancer usually develops in the endometrium (the mucous membrane inner lining) although very rare tumours do develop in the muscle of the uterus. The risk of developing cancer of the endometrium is increased in women who are older, had a late menopause, are overweight, diabetic and who have never borne children. The risk may be marginally increased for women receiving hormone treatment (Tamoxifen) for breast cancer but it is believed that the benefit gained far outweighs this very small risk.

Investigations always start with physical examination, including an internal examination. Next, the lining of the uterus will be examined under a microscope and this will confirm the diagnosis. Usually this will be done by a dilatation and curettage – a 'D&C' – at which a scraping of the lining is taken with the patient anaesthetised. Further tests include a CT or MRI scan (see 'Glossary' on pages 253–257) to check the extent of the tumour and whether the lymph glands are involved.

Treatment usually involves surgery (a total hysterectomy and removal of the ovaries and Fallopian tubes) and is often combined with radiotherapy. For older women or those who are not very fit, radiotherapy alone may be used. Radiotherapy for cancer of the endometrium may be delivered either internally or externally (see page 78), or a programme involving both methods may be used. Whichever approach is chosen, the results of treatment for early cancers are good. Hormone therapy can be used if the cancer has recurred but chemotherapy is not often used. The opportunity to talk to a counsellor should be available to women who are distressed at the thought of needing to have a hysterectomy or other treatment.

Ovaries

Ovarian cancer is one of the more common cancers in women and is the commonest cause of death for gynaecological cancers. In addition to cancer that develops in the ovaries, similar carcinomas may originate in the Fallopian tubes.

Fortunately, this cancer is rare in women under the age of 40 years. It is possibly linked to hormonal history as statistics show that it is commoner in women who are childless; taking the contraceptive pill also appears to reduce the risk. As is generally the case, there is rarely a sole cause; the hormone connection is only one element – unknown environmental factors also play a part and there is a genetic element with a link to breast cancers. Symptoms are often rather vague and there may be no symptoms at all in the early stages so that by the time the diagnosis is made cancer may well be fairly advanced. Symptoms include increasing girth and weight gain, poor appetite, nausea, vomiting and constipation and often rather imprecise abdominal discomfort. Pain and bleeding are rare.

Investigations start with a physical examination as the tumour can often be felt in the abdomen or with a combination of abdominal examination and an internal (vaginal) examination. The lump will be further assessed using ultrasound investigation and/or a CT scan. Other tests will include a chest x-ray, routine blood tests and special blood tests to look for 'tumour markers' and check hormone levels. If investigations show that there is fluid within the abdominal cavity (called ascites) then a sample of fluid may be withdrawn, under local anaesthetic, for laboratory testing. Fortunately, many suspected ovarian tumours turn out to be benign cysts.

Malignant tumours are initially treated with surgery where this is possible. Surgery involves the removal of the ovaries together with the Fallopian tubes, uterus, cervix and omentum (a fold of lining of the abdominal cavity), and the other abdominal organs are examined for possible spread of the cancer. Unfortunately, because ovarian cancer has often spread quite extensively beyond the ovary into the pelvis or throughout the abdomen when first seen, it is not always possible to remove all the tumour. Surgery is followed by chemotherapy for all but very early ovarian cancer. The drugs used to treat ovarian cancer are effective but tend to produce troublesome side effects and patients are offered support as needed during treatment.

The outlook is good for cancers found and treated early. For those people with more advanced cancer, chemotherapy is very effective in controlling the disease and giving the patient an extended period of quality life.

Reproductive system – male

Prostate

Cancer of the prostate gland is increasing in incidence, with over 15,000 new cases diagnosed annually in the UK. The annual death rate from this disease in the UK is approximately 9,600 men. Like many other cancers its cause is as yet unproven; however, also like other cancers there is a theoretical link to diet. Japanese and Chinese men are much less likely to develop prostate cancer than western men, and it may be that the high vegetable content of eastern diets may play a protective role.

Cancer of the prostate is rare in men under the age of 45 years. However, post mortem findings show an increase in incidence as age increases, with 10 to 30 per cent of men aged 50 to 60 years being affected, rising to 50 to 70 per cent of men aged 70 to 80 years. Not all these men would have been aware that they had early prostatic cancer. Fortunately, it can develop slowly or remain dormant.

Commonly, the early stages of the disease are without symptoms. If the tumour is detected early it is usually because another related problem is being investigated or it is picked up during a routine health check that includes a rectal examination. In the very early stages of the disease the man usually does not notice symptoms of obstruction similar to those of BPH (benign prostatic hyperplasia – where the gland enlarges, causing difficulty in starting to pass water). It is more usual for the disease to present at a later stage, either with pain or with symptoms of obstruction or in severe difficulty in passing urine. Other symptoms are much less specific; for example, tiredness and apathy; loss of appetite and weight loss. In 90 per cent of cases the cancer develops in other parts of the gland where it can be felt during a rectal examination or as a small, hard lump of irregular shape.

Fortunately, in at least half of the cases referred for urgent investigation the lump is benign or due to a stone. If malignancy is suspected, some or all of the following tests may be carried out: blood tests to check blood count, urea and electrolytes, prostatic acid phosphase (PAP), and prostate specific antigen (PSA). The PSA is a protein made only by prostate cells; a raised level indicates there is a high chance that prostate cancer is present. A biopsy will confirm the diagnosis. Other tests may include an ultrasound scan (which may be done with the ultrasound probe inserted into the rectum, or applied to the abdominal wall), various bone and body scans and possibly an IVP (intravenous pylegram) to view the kidneys and urinary system. The bone scan is especially important because prostate cancer frequently involves the boney skeleton and if this is the case it affects the treatment plan.

The treatment recommended will be determined by the stage of the disease at the time of diagnosis. It is common for prostate cancer to have spread beyond the prostate gland and into the surrounding tissues, the lymph nodes and bone before the patient has developed any symptoms which cause him to seek medical advice. In the less usual situation of the cancer remaining localised to the prostate gland, the individual may be offered treatment aimed at the gland itself, either by surgery or radiotherapy. If the spread is beyond the prostate gland and is causing pain then radiotherapy may be offered, often combined with hormone treatments, the aim of which is to reduce androgens (male hormones) as it is known that these promote the growth of prostate cancer cells. This can be achieved either by removing the testicles or with drugs. Hormone drug treatments are not active by mouth so they are given by injection or as a nasal spray. These hormone treatments are often extremely effective in reducing pain caused by secondary bone growths due to prostate cancer, and usually the gland itself will reduce in size improving any urinary symptoms. Radiotherapy can be used for any bone secondaries that continue to be painful.

The outlook for men with prostate cancer is quite good as hormone treatments often remain effective for many months; however, the importance of early detection (and therefore regular health checks) cannot be over-emphasised because for the few patients who present with early disease treatment may be curative.

Testicles

Unfortunately, despite increased media attention, men remain reluctant to examine their own testicles for the signs of testicular cancer – yet the number of new cases diagnosed each year in the UK exceeds 1,300. It is the third leading cause of death in younger men with the figures increasing fourfold in the last 50 years. It is rare before puberty and in old age but is the most common male cancer in younger men (age 20 to 40). The lifetime risk rate is about 1 man in 450 with the chances increasing fivefold if the man had an undescended testicle as a baby, and may be associated with other abnormalities of the genital tract. Family history plays a part as the risk rate increases to 1 in 50 if a brother has been affected. The need to raise awareness of the benefits of self-examination is vital as the disease is potentially fatal yet this is one type of cancer that can be successfully treated, especially if diagnosed early. Neither fertility nor potency are affected if one testicle remains clear.

Testicular tumours develop as a swelling of the testicles that may be painless or tender. The cancer may spread beyond the testicle to the glands in the abdomen or neck causing backache or a swelling in the neck.

Tests for testicular cancer start with examination of the testes both by feeling the shape, texture and regularity of the gland and by shining a light through the gland to see if the swelling is solid or a cyst. Ultrasound may be used if there are doubts about whether a tumour is present. A blood test to measure the levels of certain hormones (HCG and alpha-fetoprotein, which are known as 'tumour markers' and frequently produced by testicular cancers) are carried out prior to any testis being removed surgically. Subsequent treatment depends on the presence of any secondary growths and patients are very carefully assessed, as treatment with chemotherapy produces excellent results.

Urinary system

Bladder

Bladder cancer is one of the cancers that is quite often associated with a carcinogen. In the 17th century this was a chemical used in the manufacture of dyes, nowadays the likely reason will be a component of cigarette smoke. The first sign is often blood in the urine. Tests include a visual examination of the bladder (cystoscopy) using an instrument called a cystoscope, a biopsy of abnormal looking tissue, a CT scan and IV (intra-venous) examination.

Treatments depend on the stage of the cancer and will differ depending upon whether the tumour is a superficial cancer limited to the lining membrane of the bladder or an invasive cancer affecting the main bladder muscle. Early bladder cancer is usually treated by surgery, followed by close monitoring afterwards with regular cystoscopies. More invasive cancer is treated by a combination of surgery, radiotherapy and sometimes chemotherapy. Occasionally it is necessary to remove the bladder, in which case a 'false' bladder can be constructed that drains urine through a stoma onto the abdominal wall, using a piece of bowel as a conduit. The outcome of treatment depends largely on the stage at which the diagnosis was made. For superficial tumours this is good, for invasive cancers the long term chances are less predictable.

Kidneys

Cancers in this vital organ are not common. In adults, cancer of the kidney is usually diagnosed in late middle age onwards and affects men more often than women.

The early symptoms of kidney cancer may be easily missed. The presence of blood may be picked up during a routine urine test or the person may complain of discomfort in the area of the kidney caused by pressure from the developing tumour. For some people the first signs of a problem are the symptoms of cancer elsewhere, due to secondary growths. Kidney cancer often presents 'non-specifically' with general symptoms such as weight loss, fever or poor appetite.

The tests include basic investigations, examination of the urine and blood and checks on liver and kidney function. An IVP (intravenous pyelogram) is performed by taking x-rays of the kidneys and ureters after a radio-opaque dye has been injected into the vein. The dye is excreted from the kidneys and this gives information on the shape of the kidney and the collecting system, and some information on how well each kidney is functioning. Most kidney tumours can be shown on an IVP. A CT scan may be used to obtain additional information about the extent of the disease and it is sometimes performed to enable the doctor to take a tissue sample for biopsy.

If the cancer is contained within the kidney, surgery will be recommended to remove the affected kidney. The treatment of widespread secondary cancer is less satisfactory. A number of different treatments have been used over recent years including hormone treatment, chemotherapy and immunotherapy; unfortunately, none of these has a very high response rate. The outlook for patients with kidney cancer depends on the stage of the tumour at the time it is diagnosed; the prospects are clearly better if the cancer can be removed whilst it is still contained within the kidney.

Nervous system

Brain

It is important when considering brain tumours to distinguish between primary tumours that have developed from brain cells, and secondary tumours that have spread from a primary tumour elsewhere in the body. The brain is one of the commonest sites for secondary growths (metastases) to develop; primary tumours are relatively rare. Primary brain tumours tend to occur in older people, adolescents and young children (bearing in mind that all cancers in young people are rare). Little is known about the cause of these tumours with genetic factors and radiation playing a possible role. If your relative is known to have a primary cancer elsewhere in the body, it is usually fairly certain that if evidence of a brain tumour develops then this is likely to be secondary involvement, especially if several tumours are detected.

A common type of brain tumour can develop in the membrane surrounding the brain (meninges). Although the good news is that this type rarely shows signs of malignancy and is usually benign, it can be difficult to treat because of its affect on, and proximity to, vital areas of the brain. Other benign brain tumours grow in a gland found at the base of the skull (pituitary) and the nerve coverings.

The symptoms produced by brain tumours are similar whether or not they are primary or secondary growths, and depend partly on which part of the brain is involved and whether the pressure inside the head (intra-cranial pressure) is raised. If the intra-cranial pressure is

39

raised, then this may cause headaches, vomiting and disturbance of vision. The headache is often worse in the morning and may be increased by coughing or sneezing. However, headache is a common symptom and it is very rarely caused by a brain tumour and only about one-third of people with brain tumours have headaches. Quite frequently fits are the first symptom, and these may be partial fits in which only part of the body is affected by the seizure. Commonly the part affected remains weak for some hours afterwards. Neurological symptoms such as mental confusion, speech, visual and balance disturbances and behavioural changes may be evident.

Brain examination will be followed by scans to confirm that a tumour is likely and a biopsy will be performed under general anaesthetic; this is usually done if the patient is known to have a primary cancer.

Surgery is the initial treatment to remove a primary tumour if the tumour is in a part of the brain that can be operated on. If this is not possible, a biopsy will be carried out. Surgery is also used occasionally for secondary growths when there is no other spread within the body. As surgery to the brain is very critical the risks will be clearly explained to the patient and their relatives beforehand. In addition the surgeon will explain that if there is obvious evidence of a tumour when the skull is opened to take a biopsy, it is important to remove as much of the tumour as possible during the same operation.

A course of steroids is often given prior to surgery to help reduce the swelling around the tumour. In the most common forms of brain tumours (malignant gliomas), it is usually impossible to remove all the tumour so the patient is generally offered a course of radiotherapy. Chemotherapy can sometimes be used when the tumour progresses and causes further symptoms. Most patients with secondary tumours are also considered for radiotherapy. The prognosis is rarely long term for most types of malignant brain tumours so treatments are designed to ease symptoms and prevent further growth for as long as possible.

Skin

Skin cancers are common and the majority are relatively straight-forward to treat. There are two distinct types of skin cancers known as malignant melanomas and non-melanomas. The non-melanoma carcinomas are further divided into two types, named after the cells from which they originate.

- ■ **Basal cell cancers** develop from the deep layers of the skin and make up 75 per cent of skin cancers. Basal cell cancers are commonly called rodent ulcers; they virtually never spread elsewhere.
- ■ **Squamous cell cancers** form in the outer, scaly surface layer and account for 20 per cent of skin cancers. Squamous cell cancers can spread to other parts of the body, but do so very rarely.

Symptoms of non-melanoma skin cancer include small lumps and warty areas that may itch and there may be an ulcerated area that does not heal and may bleed. These cancers usually develop in areas of the body exposed to the sun such as the face, neck and backs of the hands. The non-melanoma type skin cancers carry a high success rate for detection and subsequent cure.

Treatment is primarily through surgery although radiotherapy is equally effective. The treatment suggested is partly determined by where the cancer is located and the approach that will give the best cosmetic result, especially if the lesion is on the face.

Malignant melanoma is more serious. Although it accounts for only about five per cent of skin cancers at present, the numbers detected are rising. Unfortunately, this type of cancer can be cured successfully only if it is found and treated at an early stage of its development. Usually, the changes first noticed occur in a pre-existing skin mole with alterations in shape, colour and texture; the mole may also bleed and itch. Melanomas are more commonly found in exposed parts of the body, but can develop anywhere on the skin and rarely in other sites within the body. All suspect lumps and body moles should be quickly investigated, as treatment is much more successful for early disease.

Surgery is the mainstay of treatment for melanoma. This type of skin cancer may spread to lymph nodes and other organs of the body. If this happens treatment will depend on the pattern of spread; further surgery, chemotherapy and radiotherapy may be employed.

Over-exposure to sunlight is the main cause of skin cancer; the lighter the skin colour the greater the risk. The sharp rise in skin cancers, especially malignant melanoma, is probably linked to the changes in holiday patterns with many people now taking more holidays in the sun at all times of the year. Care should be taken whenever there is exposure to sunlight as even snow and water can reflect the rays back on to the skin. The figures for melanoma show that about twice as many women as men develop the disease which may again be linked to their quest for an attractive tan.

Soft tissue sarcomas

The medical term for a malignant tumour arising in connective or soft tissue is sarcoma. Soft tissues are the parts of the body that act as supporting material – bone, muscle, fat, blood vessels (not blood itself) and the tissue surrounding nerves. This type of cancer is very rare in adults, affecting a very small number of people, about one per cent of all cancers in men and 0.6 per cent of cancers in women. However, the incidence of soft tissue cancer is greater in children, with one particular type of sarcoma affecting muscles, accounting for four to eight per cent of all childhood tumours.

Like 'cancer', 'sarcoma' is a term that covers several different types of tumour, and they are generally described according to the tissue in the body from which the tumour developed or from the cells involved.

It is not known what causes most soft tissue sarcomas to develop. Previous treatment for radiotherapy can be a factor in the development of several different types of sarcoma and certain chemicals are implicated.

The early signs and symptoms of a soft tissue cancer depend very much on where in the body it occurs. They may develop as a firm, often painless, lump or swelling in a limb, whilst a tumour that grows deep inside the body may have reached a fair size, with few obvious symptoms, before it begins to affect other organs and cause symptoms.

A number of tests involving a biopsy and scans help to make the diagnosis and estimate the extent of the tumour and possible spread to other organs. The treatment offered for sarcomas is carefully planned by a team with special experience of this rare group of tumours and usually includes a pathologist, surgeon, radiotherapist and medical oncologist. The results of treatment have improved over the years.

Skeletal system

Bone

The cancers that develop in bones are almost always secondary cancers (metastases) as primary cancers arising from bone are rare. Cancers starting in the lungs, breast and prostate commonly then spread to bone. Primary tumours that arise in bone may either develop in the bone marrow, or from the hard outer part of the bone or cartilage at the articulating joints.

The symptom first noticed when cancers involve bone is usually pain, a deep, grumbling ache that is often worse at night. The affected bone may be tender when touched, and sometimes affected bones fracture without a significant injury. If there is widespread bony involvement there is a possibility that the level of calcium in the blood will rise, and this may cause nausea, constipation and confusion. It is not uncommon for secondary involvement to be the first sign that anything is wrong, and may lead to investigations that reveal the primary site of the cancer.

Diagnosis of bone cancer is usually on x-rays or scans. The x-ray picture shows damage to the bone that is either less dense, thinner than usual, and which shows on the x-ray as a dark shadow or sometimes the bone is more dense than usual, showing light areas caused by the cancer provoking increased mineral deposits in the bone.

Bone scans are performed as in general, these are more sensitive in identifying small areas of abnormal bone than plain x-rays. A bone biopsy may be carried out to provide confirmation of the diagnosis.

Primary bone cancers are rare and the treatment will be recommended taking into account the size and spread of the tumour. It usually involves surgery in combination with chemotherapy. The good news about treatments these days is that modern surgery is far less radical than in the past with the emphasis on aiming to avoid mutilating surgery, such as amputation, whenever possible.

The treatment of secondary cancer in the bone depends on the type of primary cancer present; and may be by hormone treatment or chemotherapy. Bone pain is often very effectively treated by anti-inflammatory medication and/or radiotherapy, the latter often being given as just one treatment. If the cortex, the outer part of the bone, is very thin, surgery to strengthen the bone may be offered to avoid the complication of a spontaneous fracture, and drugs may be given to help maintain bone density.

Bone marrow (multiple myeloma)

This type of cancer is not really a bone cancer as it affects the bone marrow formed in the central cavity of bones, rather than the bone tissue itself. It develops from plasma cells (one of the many types of white blood cells) whose function is to produce antibodies (substances that neutralise toxins) as part of the body's defence against viruses and bacteria. Multiple myeloma is a rare type of cancer, commoner in older people (over 40 years) and more often diagnosed in males than females.

People with multiple myeloma produce large numbers of immature (under-developed) plasma cells in their bone marrow. As the cancer develops these affected cells spread through the bone marrow, and can spread elsewhere. The causes remain unknown; however, several industrial and environmental risk factors are being investigated. Repeated infections and drug allergies may also be linked.

Initial symptoms may include persistent pain, recurrent infections and anaemia. The abnormal plasma cells often produce excess amounts of a protein which can be detected in the blood and measured. Sometimes protein is also found in the urine. The abnormal levels of protein can damage the kidneys and cause poor kidney function. The diagnosis can often be made on a blood test but a bone marrow examination is needed to confirm the diagnosis. The mainstay of treatment is chemotherapy, aiming to destroy the abnormal plasma cells; radiotherapy is used principally to help with pain and symptom control.

Lymphatic and immune systems

Lymphomas

Cancers of the lymph system are commonly called 'lymphomas'. Like all groups of cancers there are several types with a range of names. Tumours can develop in lymphoid tissue (mainly lymph nodes/glands) found in many sites in the body. The lymphatic system consists of a mesh of very fine, thin walled tubes distributed in most tissues in the body. These little lymphatic vessels collect together to form lymphatic channels that drain into lymph nodes, and eventually form two larger lymphatic ducts that drain into the great veins. Lymph fluid is found outside blood vessels, surrounding the cells. The lymphatic system has several functions: to intercept and remove foreign material, such as bacteria, from the body and to assist with immunity through the production of antibodies. The products of inflammation and infection (bacteria and viruses) are carried to the lymph glands where they are removed, preventing the bacteria from reaching the general circulation. For example, tonsils act as a first line of defence against the germs that might cause a chest infection. Cancer cells often spread via these lymphatic vessels to the lymph nodes where they may lodge and grow.

Lymph nodes vary considerably in size, from microscopic structures lumped together to those that resemble a large bean. Well known examples of lymphoid tissue are the tonsils, the spleen, the cervical glands in the neck and the axillary glands under the armpit.

45

The cancers that develop in the lymph system may be primary or secondary depending on whether the tumour has originated in the lymph nodes or whether the cancer cells have spread there from elsewhere in the body. One type of lymphoma, Hodgkin's disease, accounts for 40 per cent of lymphomas and the remainder are collectively termed 'non-Hodgkin's lymphomas'.

Hodgkin's disease and non-Hodgkin's lymphomas

These are all cancers of the lymph tissue, so you may ask 'what's the difference?' The main difference is that Hodgkin's disease (HD) describes a set of specific symptoms named after the doctor who first described the illness in 1835; the symptoms of the other non-Hodgkin's lymphomas (NHL), although similar, are less definite in nature. Hodgkin's disease has a characteristic appearance when lymph nodes are examined under the microscope.

Identification of the various different types of non-Hodgkins lymphoma is complex and special techniques are used. Treatment is tailored to the different types of lymphoma. Lymphomas often respond very well to chemotherapy treatment; in the case of HD about 50 per cent of people diagnosed will be cured. With NHL the outlook depends on the type of lymphoma; some people are cured, in others the disease is chronic.

After a diagnosis of HD has been made according to symptoms present (enlarged glands, possible night sweats, weight loss, etc), a biopsy and various tests, the doctor will describe the extent of the disease:

- Stage I – involves a single lymph node site.
- Stage II – involves more than one lymph node site on the same side of the diaphragm.
- Stage III – involves lymph nodes on both sides of the diaphragm (including the spleen).
- Stage IV – involves one or more other organs, for example liver, bone marrow, and may or may not include glands.
- In addition, further classification is used according to the other symptoms using 'A' and 'B' sub-categories, for example IIB.

The reason for 'staging' is that treatment is determined by the extent of disease. It also allows the comparison of results of different treatments.

Non-Hodgkin's lymphomas are often generalised: this means they are often widespread involving the cells that form the blood and other tissue, such as the testes, skin and bowel. NHL appears to be on the increase and tends to affect more older people than Hodgkin's disease. It can also behave in a very aggressive manner. Like HD the non-Hodgkin's lymphomas may start with painless swelling of the lymph glands, although individuals may present with often rather vague symptoms and are only diagnosed after a number of investigations. Once the diagnosis is made, additional tests and investigations will be carried out, and these will include a biopsy that will be examined by a pathologist, often one with a special experience and interest in lymphomas.

Lymphomas are often described as low or high grade tumours, and further classified depending on the appearance of the cells and how they are arranged in the abnormal tissue.

Secondary cancer in the lymph nodes

The lymph system filters the lymphatic fluid which may pass through several lymph nodes before returning to the blood stream. This filtering system is an important role for the glands as part of the body's defence mechanism against infection; it is also this 'filtering' role that enables cancer cells to lodge and then grow in the lymph nodes. A common example of this process is the way breast cancer spreads to the lymph nodes in the armpit area. Doctors always take great care to check lymph node areas to feel for any enlargement.

Other lymphomas

Lymphomas may occur in tissues not necessarily regarded as within the lymphatic system, for example salivary glands, gastro-intestinal tract and skin. This is because nearly all tissues have some lymphoid tissue within them. Lymphomas may develop after changes have taken place in the gland following a more general illness such as auto-immune illnesses, although this is very unusual.

Leukaemia

The word 'leukaemia' triggers a great deal of fear, possibly because it can affect young children and because some types of acute leukaemia are very aggressive with a poor outlook. Leukaemia is a term that covers a number of very different conditions, they are all rare and the outlook depends on the type of leukaemia. Leukaemia means 'white blood', an early description of the disease coined because of the increased number of white cells in the blood. Leukaemia is a disease of the bone marrow, where blood cells are produced. The main characteristics of all the types include an over-production of white cells, together with enlargement of the spleen, changes in the bone marrow, marked paleness of the skin, rashes and enlargement of the lymph glands all over the body. The type of leukaemia diagnosed is named according to the type and state of white corpuscles present in the blood. The rapidly developing, acute forms are called lymphoblastic or myeloblastic leukaemia and the slow developing types are called chronic lymphatic or myeloid leukaemia. The acute forms are characterised by the proportion of immature or 'blast' cells present in the marrow and the blood. In chronic leukaemia the cells are more mature.

The acute forms are most common in young children and young adults; however, acute myeloblastic leukaemia may affect any age group. The chronic types tend to affect people over the age of 35 years and are most common in people over 60 years, but as with all cancers there are exceptions to these general guidelines. Males and females are affected equally with about 5,000 new cases diagnosed in the UK each year. The cause is unknown. Symptoms in acute cases develop rapidly, with the illness lasting only a few weeks or months. An early symptom of high fever may first be mistaken for an acute infection. The symptoms in the chronic form, as the name suggests, develop gradually and are often first noticed as enlarged glands, particularly the spleen, and as haemorrhages from different parts of the body.

The diagnosis is made by microscopic examination of a blood sample which will show an enormous increase in the number of white cells. A bone marrow examination is performed to confirm the diagnosis and the type of leukaemia present. Sometimes this can take time as special tests may be needed.

The principal treatment for the acute leukaemias is by a combination of drugs that destroy the cancerous cells whilst allowing the normal bone marrow cells to continue growing. In acute leukaemia the aim of the treatment is to induce a complete remission, in which there is no sign of the disease on a bone marrow sample. This initial treatment may be very intensive and usually the patient will need to stay in hospital whilst it is carried out. After remission has been achieved further treatment depends on the precise type of leukaemia present. In some types, maintenance treatment will be continued with chemotherapy, often over several years. For other types a bone marrow transplantation may be considered, possibly using donor marrow from a close relative, to reduce the risk of a relapse. Whatever the treatment, your relative will be closely monitored to detect relapse. If the leukaemia recurs, similar chemotherapy will be considered; however, it is harder to induce a second or subsequent remission. When this happens treatment will be directed to improve symptoms; blood transfusions and steroid therapy may be used to improve the wellbeing of the patient.

The chronic leukaemias are also treated by chemotherapy but in general the regimes used are simpler and can be undertaken at home. The emphasis is more on symptom control than trying to produce complete remission.

Unfortunately, there is no certain cure for either acute or chronic leukaemia but the outlook for both forms is changing. The chances of survival for young children have improved dramatically in recent years and the average time span from diagnosis to terminal illness for older people continues to lengthen.

For more *i*nformation

i Many books have been published about cancer. A good book shop or library will hold a range of titles and order specific books if they are not available on the shelves.

i Information can be obtained from specific cancer-related charities (listed at the end of Chapter 2) and see also the 'Useful addresses' section starting on page 258; the names of the organisations are presented in alphabetical order.

i Family Doctor Series booklets offer a wide range of titles, including *Understanding Cancer*, and are available from most chemist shops.

i PatientWise publishes a series of factsheets providing medical and health information for patients. These are available through GPs and patient information centres – ask for details at your surgery.

Conclusion

This chapter has given basic information to help you and your relative understand how cancer develops and has described in some detail the commoner cancers affecting many people today. Some of the information has been technical but knowing more about the growth and spread of tumours will help you to understand better the nature of the illness. This chapter has also looked at some of the risk factors and early detection methods as this information may provide useful advice for other family members. Being 'cancer aware' is good health sense, whatever your age. The next chapter looks in greater detail at the tests used to diagnose the type and site of the cancer and the range of treatments given as part of the management process. Future chapters will help you and your relative make positive changes to daily living and help you think about your role and responsibility as a carer.

2 Tests and treatments

In the time between visiting the GP and going to see the consultant at the hospital, people said they felt numb with fear and could not think beyond the forthcoming tests. Did you and your relative feel the same way? As you read this chapter, those early fears surrounding the diagnostic stage may now be in the past. Even if your relative has entered the treatment phase, don't be tempted to skip this chapter, as the information about tests may help you learn more about the illness and there may have been parts of the diagnostic process that you did not fully understand at the time. It isn't too late to ask why certain tests were performed and to have the results explained again if either of you need further information. The cancer team will be very aware that in times of great stress most people find it difficult to concentrate, so you may well have attended hospital appointments in a daze.

In a similar way, the wide range of treatments often cause bewilderment. You may have heard about the different treatments but are less sure why certain therapies are used with one type of cancer and not another. This chapter will help to clarify some of the tests and explain about different treatment options.

The tests – what happens and why?

As Chapter 1 explained, there are many forms of cancer according to where in the body it develops. Early investigations usually start with the consultant asking questions about any personal and family history and/or lifestyle that may have a bearing on the diagnosis. At the same visit the specialist (surgeon or medical physician) will do a physical examination. All relevant signs, symptoms and history help the doctor to get an overall picture; specific tests are then used to confirm the diagnosis and extent of disease. The particular tests subsequently performed will depend entirely on the information given by the patient and what the doctor has observed. The diagnostic process depends on the type of cancer that is suspected – tests are never done unnecessarily. Some people may attend a small local hospital whilst others have to travel further to a specialist cancer unit.

Blood tests

There are a number of blood tests used to help in the detection of a cancer but none provide an outright diagnosis, only a pointer that something is malfunctioning. Collecting a sample of blood is considered a fairly routine procedure at the start of many investigations; the blood will be used to obtain several pieces of relevant information.

- **Full blood count:** the number of cells (red, white and platelets) present in blood can indicate several facts. The haemoglobin level shows whether a person is anaemic; the white cell count gives an indication of the body's immunity system and whether it is trying to fight an infection; and the platelets are checked because they play a significant role in helping to prevent bruising and bleeding.
- **Electrolytes:** the level of certain salts in the blood (in particular sodium and potassium) is critical. Checking these levels, called an electrolyte estimation, is an important indicator that something may be wrong because an imbalance occurs quickly when the body is unwell.

- **Urea and creatinine:** the levels are measured to estimate the function of the kidneys.
- **Liver function tests:** the liver is responsible for converting broken-down foodstuffs into materials essential for other body actions. The level of protein and certain enzymes indicate whether the liver is working correctly and efficiently.
- **Special blood tests** are performed when certain types of cancer are suspected. The detection of cancers that form in the reproductive tissue (testes and ovaries) is one example. The laboratory investigation checks for a substance called alpha-fetoprotein because of its connection with germ cell tissue; levels of this substance are also raised during pregnancy. This is called a **serum marker** and for some cancers the level of the marker can give useful information about how the cancer is responding to treatment.

Biopsy

The presence and type of cancer can usually be decided by looking at some tissue under a microscope. This is one of the starting (and confirming) points for diagnosis. The word 'biopsy' literally means 'the removal and examination of tissue from the living body for diagnostic purposes' (*Black's Medical Dictionary*). In a nutshell this is exactly what happens. A small piece of the tumour is removed and sent to the laboratory for diagnosis. It is possible that the suspected tissue will be removed during the first visit to the hospital but, however urgent the need for diagnostic action, the decision about how and when to perform a biopsy will depend entirely on the site of the lump.

In many cases a small operation is performed at an outpatient clinic or day surgery centre. The patient is given a local anaesthetic to freeze the area or a general anaesthetic to put them temporarily to sleep so that the tissue can be removed without discomfort. Fortunately, the need for a general anaesthetic is rarer now that special techniques allow the precise removal of tissue from deep inside the body without using traditional surgery; for example, tissue can be taken from the liver through a needle insertion. Occasionally the material removed is in fluid form or a scraping of cells is smeared on to a glass slide, rather than solid tissue. Sometimes the person is asked to stay in hospital for a longer period in case the circumstances make it necessary to perform an immediate operation. Often a surgeon will request permission to remove the tumour completely when he or she gets a clearer internal view; a piece of the removed tissue will be sent to the laboratory. To perform a biopsy and then have to re-open the operation site following a positive diagnosis is not in the best interest of the patient. If there is any chance that the surgeon may need to make this decision, the options will be explained clearly to the patient and their relatives beforehand.

Diagnosis often takes a week or two and the results may be sent to your relative's GP who will explain the findings and make sure that everyone understands what will happen next. Alternatively, an appointment may be made at the hospital so that the results of the biopsy can be given and treatment discussed.

Fibreoptic endoscopy

This test may sound very technical but it is simply a description of 'what happens and how'. A fibreoptic endoscopy is an investigation that enables a specialist to look into a hollow body cavity using an instrument called an endoscope. The device is fitted with a source of cold light that passes down a bundle of quartz fibres, sometimes up to 20,000 fibres at a time. Despite the large numbers of fibres carried by the tube it is very narrow and extremely flexible.

The use of this technique has radically changed the way that doctors can view parts of the body that used to be inaccessible without a minor operation. The endoscope is manipulated from the outside so that the operator can see and do whatever is needed. The finger-tip controls enable the surgeon to remove mucus or a small piece of tissue for biopsy and the image is passed back to the outside by reflected light. Usually the examination can be done easily with a mild sedative and local anaesthetic.

This technique is commonly used in the following situations:

- A **bronchoscopy** to examine the airways leading to and directly into the lungs with the tube being passed through the nose.
- An **oesophagoscopy**, **gastroscopy** and **duodenoscopy** to examine a particular part of the upper gastro-intestinal tract, the tube leading to and into the stomach from the mouth.
- A **colonoscopy** to check the upper part of the intestinal tract, above the rectum, from the anal end. The lower part of the bowel (the rectum) is generally examined manually by the doctor with an inserted finger and visually using a smooth, rigid metal instrument. This check is called a **sigmoidoscopy**.
- A **cystoscopy** to examine the tube leading from the bladder (urethra) and the bladder itself. A light general anaesthetic may be given to avoid undue discomfort.

X-rays

- **Basic x-ray** Most people are familiar with a general x-ray. Short rays capable of penetrating soft tissue, such as muscle and fat, are beamed onto a photographic plate, thus giving a picture of what lies under the surface skin. Hard tissue (bone) stops the progress of the ray and so it looks denser and stands out against the soft tissue. X-ray tests can be used to outline the shape of tumours in the digestive tract and more sophisticated procedures have been developed to assist in diagnosis and screening and allow much more detail to be seen (see 'Mammogram' and 'Scans' below).
- **Barium meal** This x-ray involves swallowing a substance, often barium sulphate, that creates a contrast picture on the photographic film. The patient may be asked to fast overnight to ensure the digestive tract is relatively empty. Immediately prior to the x-ray procedure, a cupful of barium is swallowed and the patient lies on a couch. The x-ray pictures are taken continuously whilst linked to a TV monitor. The radiographer (the person trained to operate the x-ray machine) moves the patient into several positions to give a range of pictures from different angles. The film is then developed and the frames

separated for closer inspection. The test may sound unpleasant but it is not painful.

■ **Barium enema** This special x-ray is identical to the barium meal, but taken from the reverse end of the digestive tract. The bowel must be completely empty so clear directions will be given to the patient beforehand about dietary control and the use of laxatives. The barium fluid, together with air, is inserted into the bowel via a tube and the x-ray pictures taken as required. The test can cause discomfort and a bloated feeling – gas will continue to escape after the test is completed!

■ **Intravenous urogram (sometimes called a 'pyelogram' or IVP)** This test is designed to look at the kidneys and the tubes leading from the kidneys that carry urine down to the bladder (ureters). A special dye, visible on x-ray, is injected into a vein and is photographed as it makes its way through the drainage system via the kidneys. This procedure gives a clear picture of the shape, position and structure of the kidneys and ureters, but it does have some disadvantages – it's quite a lengthy process and the dye may cause the patient's skin to look greenish in colour for a short while.

■ **Cholecystogram** This test is similar to an IVP but is designed to check the function and shape of the liver, bile duct and gall bladder. The radio-opaque dye is usually given by mouth.

■ **Arteriogram, venogram and lymphogram** These tests use radio-opaque dyes to examine arteries, veins and the lymph system.

■ **Mammogram** This x-ray is best known for its preventative screening function rather than as a pure detection tool (see page 14). The pictures are examined for signs of cancer or other abnormalities that show up before they can be felt. All women, whatever their age, should be aware of any changes in their breasts (see page 15 for self-examination guidelines).

Scans

Scanning is a relatively new procedure compared with traditional x-rays and one that is much more exact. Scans are used to give the cancer team a picture of the size, position and shape of the tumour (rather than a means of diagnosis) so that subsequent scans can be taken to monitor the effects of treatment.

The scanning process uses a number of different techniques. Computed tomography (CT) and magnetic resonance imaging (MRI) scanning use a similar manoeuvre where the whole body, or a smaller section, is moved slowly through a tunnel-shaped cavity whilst 'pictures' are taken. Most modern machines require the patient to be very still (with breath held) for only a few seconds, although the process can hold fears for people who are concerned about being shut into a narrow space. In reality, many people are relieved that it was less frightening than they had imagined. The staff operating the equipment are very supportive and always present if help is needed. The different scanning processes include:

- **Radioactive isotope scan (sometimes called nuclear medicine)** In this test, tiny quantities of radioactive material called isotopes are used to detect abnormalities. The process works because many substances found naturally in the body, such as iodine, can be used to carry radioactive material which emits radiation. The isotope, together with its carrier, is introduced by an appropriate method (eg via a vein) and after a short while the radiation given off is scanned by a special camera. The distribution of radiation is then measured and recorded to give a visual plot indicating high and low spots. It is also used to view changes in bone tissue where secondary cancer may have formed. The technique requires special equipment so patients may be asked to travel to a cancer centre for the test. Isotope testing is also used in other forms of diagnostic medicine; for example, to measure the action of the thyroid gland.
- **Ultrasound (ultrasonic) scan** This is a test most commonly associated with pregnancy; however, it is also used as a way of examining many other organs. Ultrasound has several advantages: it is non-invasive, quick, inexpensive, versatile and harmless so it can be repeated as often as necessary. It is rapidly replacing other investigative processes such as radiography and isotope scanning (see above). Ultrasound is so refined that very small lumps can be detected and the operator can carry out a needle biopsy using ultrasound as a guide. In particular,

organs deep in the abdomen, the breasts and testicles can be checked by ultrasound technique with little discomfort. Water soluble oil is spread over the area to be examined to help the instrument make good contact with the skin. Sound waves that move at frequencies far above the level heard by the human ear (15 kilocycles per second) are bounced from a scanning head through the body tissue (via body fluids) and back to their source. The head of the instrument is moved steadily over the surface and the picture is transmitted back to the analyser which converts electronic signals into live pictures on a screen. The still pictures can be printed for future examination.

■ **Computed tomography (CT)** This is a special x-ray technique that enables clearly focused images to be taken in a wafer-thin 'slice' showing the structures present there. Thousands of readings are taken in very small slices, half to one centimetre apart, so that the resulting picture (a tomograph) can be viewed as a series of cross sections of the body. X-rays are beamed across the tunnel where the patient is lying and through the patient to be picked up by special sensors. The information is fed into a computer that constructs a picture of what is present within each body slice photographed. The tomograph gives a valuable image of how a tumour mass may be distorting an organ or where the lump is of a different density to the surrounding tissue. Occasionally, special x-ray-sensitive dyes and fluids are inserted or swallowed to intensify the image. The technique was first introduced in 1977 and is now accepted as a regular part of cancer care.

■ **Magnetic resonance imaging (MRI)** This is another technique that uses computers combined with powerful energy waves to produce a picture of a body area. In this procedure radio waves (instead of x-rays) are intermittently beamed at the body within a strong magnetic field causing a certain alignment of body cells (atomic nuclei) in the direction of the field. The technique employs the knowledge that differing structures of tissues give off different vibratory energy signals. These signals are then built up by the computer to form a picture of the tissue being investigated in any body plane, similar to CT. However, although MRI is very useful in neurological examinations, it is less useful in cancer detection or continuing care because the cancerous tumour may not easily be separated visually from the surrounding healthy tissue. The process may take some time, and can be very noisy.

A diagnosis has been made – what happens now?

John, a doctor

'A diagnosis of cancer means just that – a form of cancer has been found somewhere in the body. A diagnosis of cancer is not an immediate death sentence. It is possible that your relative's life will end sooner than you had imagined but it is also possible that the cancer will be cured or a lengthy period of remission will give them many more years of life.'

This is a difficult time and you may feel that you are walking in a dream. People in shock rarely absorb everything at once so don't be worried about asking questions over again. The medical team are aware of your distress so no one will mind repeating a piece of information. Be sure that your relative is clear about the next stages, especially if decisions have to be made about treatment. You can help by listening carefully on their behalf and taking notes if this would help you remember words and instructions. Later, in a quieter moment, you can both recall what you heard and help each other to remember what information was given. Try not to feel rushed. Hospital clinics and doctors' surgeries are not peaceful places and waiting around can make you feel panicky so that you want to get home as quickly as possible. Take your time and don't let the pressures of busy staff get to you.

Filling the time gap – from diagnosis to treatment

The diagnosis is made using information gathered from three main sources: the list of symptoms described by your relative; the relevant details from their medical history; and the results of the tests. From this parcel of facts the doctor will put together a programme of treatment. Waiting for the test results may have felt like forever; equally frustrating is the wait before treatment commences. Rest assured, most cancers do not grow so quickly that a short delay at this stage will have a serious long-term effect. Use the time delay positively to help support your relative and do some short term planning. For example, you may need to make arrangements for care in the home if your relative is too frail to be left alone; re-arrange your work schedule to accompany your relative to hospital for chemotherapy treatment; and you could spend time building up your mental reserves for the tiring time ahead. Perhaps you (and your relative) would find relief by talking to someone outside the immediate family circle. Sharing your feelings with a person who has no emotional links with your situation can provide a welcome release from tension – someone from one of the cancer charities may be the right person to fulfil this supporting role (see pages 258–274 for national helpline details). Church leaders of any denomination are also willing to spend time with patients and families at this time even if the person does not have a direct religious need. And, finally, you could introduce some form of relaxing therapy. Aromatherapy, reflexology and Bach Flower remedies (see Chapter 8, 'Managing stress') are well-established complementary therapies – a session with a trained therapist may help take your mind off the immediate problem.

Look upon the illness as a journey without a clearly defined map of the route and an unknown destination. At several points along the road you will need to stop and support your relative whilst serious decisions are made about future direction. When you reach these 'crossroads', perhaps involving treatment options or terminal care, a team of professional people will be there to help you take the next steps but the final decisions always lie with the person who is ill, and their family if they are not able to make such decisions. This analogy is a way of illustrating that every family affected by cancer follows a similar, unfamiliar path with similar experiences and anxieties.

Understanding treatments

In the same way that there are lots of tests to help detect cancer, so there are also several different kinds of treatments. The choices were outlined briefly in Chapter 1; this chapter will look at each type in greater detail. Cancer treatment frequently causes confusion because of the range of therapies. Most people think of surgery as the probable starting point for treatment but are less sure about what follows and why one patient is given one combination and another patient gets something different. Common questions cover 'How do doctors decide? and, 'How much say does the patient have in this decision?' The basic answers lie ahead; however, if you have specific questions about your relative's treatment, you must ask the cancer team direct.

Lisa, a doctor

'Whatever stage your relative is at and whichever mixture is now being offered or was given, you can be sure that it is or was the best combination for your relative's particular type of cancer.'

Cancer treatment choices depend on many factors that are discussed with the patient, and with his or her family if he or she wishes, as part of the decision-making process. Some older patients with dementia may not be capable of making an independent decision. The factors taken into account include:

- the age and general health of the patient;
- the organ and cells that the cancer has grown from;
- the size and extent of the tumour;

- whether the tumour has spread to other organs;
- whether it is important to try to preserve fertility;
- which facilities and treatments are readily available within reasonable travelling time;
- personal preference of the patient.

After treatment options have been explained, it is quite in order for your relative to ask the doctor for time to think things over. A day or so spent discussing the proposed treatment programme will make little difference to the outcome and will enable all the relevant people to feel that they have played a part in making the decision. Being involved brings back a sense of control, particularly if there is a choice about where to go for treatment. Everyone must be absolutely sure that starting on a course of exhausting treatment (surgery and/or chemotherapy) is what the patient really wants and that they know what the alternatives are. The option to decline treatment should never be overlooked or disregarded in the desire to try to bring about a cure.

John, a doctor

'To say "no" in the face of positive talk by hospital staff and the love and optimism of close family and friends is a very brave decision for a patient to make. But it may be the route that some people wish to consider, especially if they feel too frail or their cancer is too advanced to undergo surgery. For such people I offer counselling and give a clear explanation of what palliative care can offer, as I believe that such information is an important element in helping them make their choice.

'Equally, it can be difficult to understand why, sometimes, no treatment is offered. When this happens it is usually because your relative has a cancer that is not curable and so any treatment is aimed at relieving symptoms. If your relative has no symptoms, or if they are unlikely to be relieved by anticancer treatment, then the best option is often to "watch and wait".'

Surgery

Removal of the cancerous lump is the main aim of surgery and is probably the first thought that people seize upon – to take away this alien 'thing' as soon as possible. People say 'my body is being invaded', 'I am playing host to an uninvited guest' and 'I find it difficult to feel at ease with this intruder'. These are age-old sentiments and surgery has been the primary treatment for cancer as long as mankind has kept medical records, albeit in a crude form. The Greeks and Romans recognised cancer as a threat to life and performed primitive surgery in an attempt to cure. Fortunately, medical knowledge has developed somewhat, particularly the discovery of anaesthetics and improved hygiene. The proficiency of surgical techniques now makes it possible for surgery be used to treat almost every cancer. If surgery is deemed not to be appropriate for your relative it will be for a very valid reason: maybe their health is too frail; the tumour is too advanced to be removed, or because other treatments are more fitting.

Margaret

'My granddaughter told my husband to learn to accept his cancer when he couldn't have surgery. That suggestion felt wrong at first but gradually he came to terms with having it inside him.'

For most people, surgery plays a role in several stages of cancer management:

- **Diagnosis** (see 'Biopsy', page 53).
- **Treatment** Ideally, the prime aim of any surgical operation is the complete removal of the tumour, whilst it is contained within an organ; however, how much of the cancerous tissue can be removed will not be entirely known until the area is visible. Once the cancer is exposed the surgeon tries to remove all the obvious cancerous growth and the surrounding tissue where the malignant

cells might have spread. If the operation is done at an early stage the chances of secondary growths appearing are greatly reduced and, with good fortune, it may never develop again elsewhere.

■ **Reconstruction** Techniques are now very sophisticated so that many operations can be performed that were impossible a few years ago. For example, plastic surgery is used very effectively to rebuild areas and restore appearance in breast or facial surgery (see page 102).

■ **Palliation** In this procedure, surgery is used to ease discomfort when it is no longer possible to bring about a cure. An example is where a cancer in the colon is too advanced to be removed completely but is causing an obstruction to the digestive system. Bypassing the tumour improves the situation and gives the person a better quality of life even though the improvement may be only temporary.

Surgical techniques

There are several surgical procedures open to the surgeon. The method chosen will depend on factors similar to those used to decide treatment: the position of the tumour, the general health and age of the patient and, importantly, which technique gives the best results. If your relative has undergone surgery (or is waiting for a date) it is likely that one of the following methods will have been explained to you. If you are unclear about the operation and would like more detailed explanation, do ask for help.

Traditional surgery, where an extensive area of the body surface is opened in order to view or remove a major organ, is necessary for most cancers. Examples include removal of a section of bowel to create a colostomy; removal of a breast or a piece of skull bone to excise a brain tumour.

Less invasive surgery may be done to assess the stage of a cancer and to decide if it is appropriate to go ahead with a major operation.

Other recent advances in surgery you may have heard about, such as 'micro', 'keyhole' and 'laser' surgery, are less likely to be used for cancer treatment.

Procedures before surgery

Cancer treatment is performed on a day patient or an in-patient basis, depending on the nature of the surgery and the length of time that it takes to carry out the operation. Day patients are asked to arrive at the day hospital an hour or so beforehand; in-patients are usually admitted to a ward the day before. Both procedures allow sufficient time for a clear explanation about the forthcoming anaesthetic and operation and to carry out necessary tests and checks. These cover:

- a general health check, including temperature, blood pressure, etc;
- suitability to receive an anaesthetic (checking that the person is free from chest infection, for example);
- possible urine test;
- possible blood samples, perhaps to check blood group and haemoglobin levels;
- signing the consent form for the operation and anaesthetic.

On the day of the surgery no food or drink must be taken for several hours prior to the operation. Fortunately, modern anaesthetics are much improved so nowadays patients are less likely to suffer nausea and sickness after surgery. You will be given clear instructions beforehand about what to do if your relative is a day patient.

If a general anaesthetic is to be given, shortly before the journey to the operating theatre special pre-medication is usually given either as an injection or a tablet to induce drowsiness; the drugs cause deep relaxation without putting the patient to sleep. In the anaesthetic room the patient is already sedated but still able to respond to instructions. Immediately prior to the main anaesthetic, an injection is given into a vein that brings about instant sleep and the full anaesthetic is then administered. At no time will the patient feel any discomfort or pain and they will not be wheeled into the operating theatre until the anaesthetist is sure they are completely unconscious.

Surgery may also be carried out under local anaesthetic or epidural (spinal) analgesia, which is carried out with the patient sedated, but awake. A special technique will be chosen to make sure that the part of the body being operated on is quite numb so that no pain is felt but your relative will be aware of what is happening at the time.

After the operation

After the operation your relative will spend some time in a special room called a recovery area where specially trained nurses closely monitor a patient whilst they come around from the anaesthetic. Once consciousness is regained and the anaesthetist is satisfied that there are no immediate problems from the anaesthetic, the patient is wheeled back to the ward on a trolley, accompanied by trained attendants; your relative will remain very sleepy at this stage.

How long your relative stays in hospital after the operation will depend on how well they recover in the immediate post-operative period and on the type of operation they have received. Day patients who have had a small lump removed will almost certainly be able to go home within a few hours. Same-day surgery is now very common and evidence over recent years has shown that patients who are discharged quickly make a very rapid recovery, with no obvious ill effects.

Your relative will be encouraged to get up and move about shortly after the operation to avoid the risks associated with post-operative bed rest. The main problems that occurred post-operatively in the past – blood clots developing in the veins of the legs, chest infections and wound infections – are now less common due to enormous advances in post-operative care. Patients are advised individually about such things as diet, exercise and returning to work. The specialist management and advice necessary after certain tests, treatments and operations (stoma care, cosmetic surgery, breast prosthesis, wigs, etc) are covered in Chapter 3. If your relative is recovering from a specific operation they will be given very careful instructions by the medical staff about how to deal with their particular condition. If either you or your relative is unsure about the information given by the ward staff, do ask for a clear explanation – maybe a leaflet will be available that you can take home and read when you feel less anxious. Before your relative is discharged the next stage of the treatment will undoubtedly be discussed, if any is required, and arrangements made for a follow-up visit.

Convalescence

Time spent 'convalescing' in the old-fashioned sense, where a patient went to a special home to recover, is rarely suggested these days, although some nursing homes do offer this facility. However, the need for time spent in convalescence is still very important after an operation, particularly if the surgery was extensive. Most patients are encouraged to be up and about as soon as is practical after an operation but that does not mean your relative can take up life exactly where they left off prior to their diagnosis. No person should expect to jump up like a 'spring chicken' immediately after surgery, whatever their age or illness! Patients with cancer are no exception; they may continue to feel poorly for a while, especially if other forms of treatment commence shortly after the operation.

The best advice to your relative is to be as active as they feel able and to convalesce in the traditional way by resting, relaxing and gradually increasing their daily activities without over-taxing their body. You can help by being supportive and taking care of their everyday affairs until they slip back into a normal routine. It will help them to know that you (or family members) are around to provide assistance and maybe fend off over-eager acquaintances – but do guard against being too protective.

Chemotherapy

Surgery and radiotherapy deal with cancers directly at the site of the tumour; chemotherapy differs in that it is a generalised treatment that affects the whole body. By the nature of the disease, cancer almost invariably spreads to other organs unless the rogue cells are destroyed, so it is necessary where possible to kill any cancer cells before they develop elsewhere into secondary cancers. Chemotherapy can also be used where the cancer has already spread to other sites in the body as chemotherapy drugs reach all the areas involved. Chemotherapy is offered to combat a range of cancers although it is not an effective treatment in all cancers. In particular, it is used in the treatment of acute leukaemia, lymphomas, childhood and adult cancers. The therapy may be given in combination with surgery and/or radiotherapy; the exact programme will be aimed at achieving the best results.

The name chemotherapy means 'treatment with chemicals' – drugs that actively destroy body cells. In cancer treatment, the term applies to drugs that are capable of damaging cancer cells. Strictly speaking, all drug treatments (including hormone and immuno-therapy described below) are drug therapies, but in medical language the term 'chemotherapy' refers only to the special cytotoxic drugs used for cancer treatment. Cytotoxic drugs work by damaging all cells – cancerous and normal. They are given in such a way that the damage to the cancer cells is maximised and the damage to normal cells is minimised. The treatment is tailored to reduce, as far as possible, the side effects caused by the drugs and the damage to normal tissue.

Which drugs are used?

There are several types of cytotoxic drugs in use, often given in combinations, according to the type of cancer. The information given below lists a few examples only, there are a number of different drugs in each category.

■ The **alkylating agents** work by attacking DNA (the blueprint information for the cell) thus interfering with cell reproduction; examples of drugs include mustine and ifosfamide.
■ The **cytotoxic antibiotics** used primarily in the treatment of acute leukaemia and lymphomas include doxorubicin and bleomycin.

- The **antimetabolites** combine with vital enzyme systems of the cell to prevent normal cell division. An enzyme is a chemical produced naturally by the body to trigger an important body process. Drugs used are fluorouracil and methotrexate.
- The **vinca alkaloid group** of drugs include vinchristine and vinblastine, often used to treat lymphomas and leukaemias.

The source of the drugs

Scientists are working continually to develop new drug treatments and improve existing drugs. The raw materials from which the drugs are derived come mainly from natural substances collected all over the world; for example, plants and fungus from the rain forests, algae from water and metal derivatives. Some drugs have been found because of a direct search by pharmaceutical companies for likely substances; others are discovered more by chance when researchers come across a promising candidate whilst doing other experiments. The drug doxorubicin (mentioned above) was discovered in Northern Italy from a fungus taken from the ruins of a medieval tower. This drug is now widely used in the treatment of non-Hodgkin's lymphomas.

Chemotherapy treatments are chosen because:

- certain cancers respond to some drugs and not others;
- the route by which the drugs are given will be decided on the physical characteristics of the drug and how it is handled by the body;
- some drugs are better taken as pills by mouth whilst others must be injected;
- some drugs cause damage to the tissues if given in their pure form so they must be diluted considerably and run into the body through a fast-flowing intravenous drip;
- some drugs work best in high concentrations so they are injected directly into the site of the cancer.

The commonest route is by intravenous injection, usually given via a drip, at a cancer day centre. Some patients taking oral drugs can self-manage the treatment at home; whilst a small number of people require hospital admission where they can be carefully monitored.

The drugs are given as a complete course over a variable time period. The schedules usually take from one to several days, repeated at intervals over one to four weeks, for up to eight cycles. Occasionally, low doses are given continuously for a period lasting many weeks. If this regime is the most suitable, the patient will be fitted with a special pump connected to a plastic tube running into the wall of the chest through which the drug seeps at a steady rate. The person is usually well enough to carry out normal activities with the pump strapped to their body. A Hickman line (see page 207) is one example of such a system.

Adjusting to the treatment

Patients who attend cancer centres soon get into the routine and some people manage to fit attendance at the out-patient clinic around their normal daily life. How well or poorly a person feels depends largely on their age and what combination of drugs they are being given, and, to a small degree, their personal approach to the treatment. There are some publicised cases of well-known people undergoing cancer treatment whilst still continuing to work. Patients receiving small doses of drugs in tablet form (for example, for low-grade non-Hodgkin's lymphomas) may respond well to such treatment. But for most people having chemotherapy and continuing to lead a busy life will simply not be an option; getting themselves through the treatment period will be about as much as they can manage. This is not the time for heroics. It is likely that your relative will need considerable physical and emotional support whilst receiving chemotherapy.

Side effects

Lisa, a doctor

'When chemotherapy was first developed, the early drugs in use had very unpleasant side effects. The patients suffered severe nausea and vomiting shortly after being given the medication but the effects on the cancers (especially lymphomas and leukaemias) was so amazing that it was considered essential to carry on. Chemotherapy for those first patients must have been very hard to endure. The great news for patients nowadays is that modern cytotoxic treatment is radically different than it was a decade or so ago. Almost every aspect of care is changing and developing; the drugs in common use cause fewer side effects and are more effective; other medication is available to counter the negative characteristics; and the long-term prospects for recovery have improved.'

Side effects that remain are largely related to the action of the drugs that, unfortunately, harm normal cells as well as destroying malignant cells. The cells most affected are those that are renewed most often; for example, the skin and hair follicle cells and the lining of the gut. But unlike cancerous cells, the healthy cells grow again so the damage is repairable. It may feel unbearable for your relative at the time but do reassure them, it does get better rapidly.

There are a number of short- and long-term side effects, many of which can be controlled:

Nausea and vomiting is now much reduced thanks to the development of anti-emetic (sickness-reducing) drugs. The nausea is caused by the cytotoxic drugs affecting the stomach lining and the area of the brain that controls vomiting – similar to the effects of travel sickness. It is rare for a patient on chemotherapy to have very troublesome nausea and vomiting as it can be almost totally controlled.

Hair loss remains a problem for many people depending on the type of drug they are prescribed. Loss varies from slight thinning of the hair to a total loss in all areas of the body where hair grows. Of course, the loss of scalp hair is the most noticeable effect and the most distressing for patients, but the effect is usually very temporary – as soon as treatment ends the hair begins to grow again. In the meantime, female patients can cover their head with a hat, scarf or wig. A covering helps to disguise the bald patches making this visible sign of chemotherapy less noticeable and it helps to keep the head warm. For male patients, hair loss is less obvious and even fashionable but a hat may be welcome to keep out the cold. Reduction of hair loss can be achieved when taking some cytotoxic drugs by chilling the scalp during treatment; the cooling reduces the damage to the hair roots. Clinic staff will be able to give advice on these matters.

Fiona, cancer centre nurse

'The appearance of new growth can be quite exciting so if your relative wishes you could hold a mirror to help them to see the first, silky hair sprouts. The hair re-grows at a normal rate and initially it may be more curly due to root damage. Encourage your relative to have their hair styled regularly as short hair looks good if it is shaped well to the contours of the head. Many hairdressers are used to cutting hair for people after chemotherapy so they will be very sympathetic and some salons provide a home service.' *(For more tips on hair care, see page 108.)*

Bone marrow damage takes place because the developing blood cells (red cells, white cells and platelets – see 'Glossary' on pages 253–257) forming in the bone marrow are very sensitive to the cytotoxic drugs. The blood count is monitored very closely throughout chemotherapy and the doses adjusted accordingly. The reduction in cell numbers can have different effects on the patient: loss of red cells causes anaemia; loss of white cells causes a lowered resistance to infection and loss of platelets causes bruising and bleeding into the tissues. If levels become too low, blood and platelet transfusions can be given and injections of growth factors can improve the white cell count.

Diarrhoea is a side effect of some chemotherapy drugs. Although loose bowels are unpleasant, the problem can easily be remedied using basic anti-diarrhoea products purchased at any high street pharmacy. The nurse doing the health check at the chemotherapy clinic will advise your relative, but if a bout of diarrhoea starts it does need swift attention. All pharmacists are trained to give professional advice; be sure to tell them that chemotherapy drugs might be causing the problem. If the diarrhoea attack is severe the oncologist will probably suggest a mini-break in the treatment.

Fertility may be affected for both male and female patients. Male sperm count and female ovulation are reduced temporarily or permanently by some cytotoxic drugs. For older patients this rarely presents a problem (unless an older man wishes to remain fertile). For younger patients it may be of considerable importance so the issue should be clearly discussed before starting treatment. A male patient can be given the opportunity to bank sperm samples and female patients can ask to have their ova frozen for later use. The rules on storage of female eggs are becoming less strict and the techniques for post-cancer fertilisation are improving. Counselling is available for patients who have been made infertile by chemotherapy to help them overcome this loss. Women who experience a premature menopause causing unwelcome hormone-induced symptoms can ask to be given replacement therapy. For patients who remain sexually active and fertile during chemotherapy (given that energy levels may be noticeably reduced) it is advisable that a suitable form of contraception is used during and after the treatment. It would be unwise to conceive a child whilst the effects of chemotherapy are still present. For more information about giving and receiving sexual pleasure in the time surrounding the illness, see page 125.

A **sore mouth and mouth ulcers** can be a problem. Many centres provide patients with a mouthwash to use after meals, but if your relative has not been offered this, the local pharmacy will recommend a suitable product.

If **dry and itchy skin** is causing irritation, gently massage with appropriate lotions or oils such as baby oil, but avoid some aromatherapy oils without seeking advice from a trained therapist as they can have powerful effects that may interfere with other drugs (see page 242).

Some drugs damage the nerves producing **pins and needles**, **numbness** or **pain** in the hands or feet. This is usually temporary.

Pre-treatment checks

Monitoring procedures for all possible side effects will be a regular pre-therapy check at out-patient visits. The whole routine is designed to be as relaxed as possible; however, be prepared for long waits because it takes time to do the necessary tests and read the results before the dose for that session can be prescribed. A blood test is done before each treatment to check blood count levels. Patients are checked over by a specially trained nurse and asked to answer questions using a standard questionnaire. Once again, this is not a time for heroics; if your relative is feeling poorly it is important to tell the medical team so that where possible the problem can be addressed. Whilst the treatment is being given your relative will sit in a comfortable armchair or lie on a bed depending on how long it takes for the drip to run through and how well they feel.

Molly, cancer centre nurse

'Most cancer centres provide patients with a booklet that outlines the treatment regime. It gives basic information about the drugs being used; explains the risk of side effects and gives clear advice about what to do if the patient or carers are worried. It is usually possible for patients to telephone for help at any time of the day or night as experienced cancer team members are on duty at all times.'

> ### *Nan, a relative*
>
> 'I telephoned at 2.00am because my mother was feeling poorly and had got herself into a state. Even in the middle of the night a nurse listened to my problem and suggested how to settle her down.'

Taking precautions to avoid infection

During the treatment period it is advisable to avoid public places (and friends or relatives who are unwell), especially when colds and influenza germs are in the air. Chemotherapy causes a lowered resistance to infection so be aware of the dangers and take a few basic precautions to avoid additional ill health. Keep a watchful eye on your relative generally for the early warning signs that an infection is brewing. The most obvious symptoms are a raised temperature often coupled with a sore throat or feeling generally unwell. If these are evident, ask your relative's GP for advice as it is important to take action quickly, especially if the blood count is low. If your relative is recovering from surgery, check out the operation site to ensure the scar is healing well.

The future

Fortunately, research continues to progress and newer types of therapies replace outdated and less effective methods. Patients are finding that treatment regimes are less awesome than they had imagined. This is good news and such welcome tidings should be broadcast widely. There is no doubt that chemotherapy is an ordeal, for which the love and support of families and professional staff is vital; however, a positive message about chemotherapy from those who know and have recovered could help other patients feel less fearful and start their therapy with a resolute attitude.

Radiotherapy

Radiotherapy is a form of treatment using radiation. The doses are accurately calculated and directed very precisely at the site of the cancer. There is no danger that the whole body could be made radioactive. The history of the treatment began at the end of the nineteenth century when a German scientist showed that x-rays could penetrate objects. Shortly after his discovery French doctors, Pierre and Marie Curie, detected radium. It was the combination of these discoveries that led to present-day radiotherapy. Its use today is largely confined to cancer medicine, to reduce and control the size and growth rate of tumours.

Radiation is produced by beaming electrons at a metal plate where, upon impact, the energy they carry is converted into x-rays, or by using a radioactive substance that emits gamma rays of an appropriate energy. The energy of the x-rays can be modified by the energy of the electron beam as it hits the plate. The higher the energy of the resulting x-rays, the greater the depth the energy is deposited within the tissues of the body, whilst less radiation is absorbed by the more superficial tissues and skin. The radiation causes damage to the DNA (the 'blueprint' information held in each cell) affecting the cell's ability to reproduce itself. The cell struggles to continue dividing as part of its growth process but eventually dies. The technology of radiotherapy is now so well developed that maximum doses of rays can be directed at malignant cells whilst minimising damage to surrounding healthy tissue. It is possible that some normal tissue will be irradiated but, as with chemotherapy damage, the healthy tissue is able to re-grow without lasting injury. Treatment is given in small, daily doses calculated to harm the cancerous cells but allow the healthy cells to recover.

When is radiotherapy given?

Radiation is used in several ways. It can be given as the sole means of treatment with the hope that the cancer will be cured, particularly where an operation causes an unacceptable loss of function or disfigurement. For example, in early cancer of the larynx (voice box), radiotherapy allows the individual to keep their voice, whereas surgery involves removal of the larynx and therefore loss of the voice.

Often radiotherapy is combined with other treatment such as surgery or chemotherapy, either to 'shrink' a tumour so that surgery can take place with a lesser operation, or following surgery if there is concern that some cancer cells have been left behind in the 'tumour bed'. Radiation treatment may follow after chemotherapy has been effective when it can be used to treat any residual tumour cells that may remain.

Radiotherapy can also be used as a palliative treatment to help troublesome symptoms. This method is the most widely used as it provides relief of symptoms when a total cure is not possible. Radiotherapy can be given to reduce the size of the tumour, giving swift relief in a number of situations; for example, when the tumour is growing close to bones and nerves or when it is causing an obstruction by pressing on soft tissue. Low doses are given and can be repeated whenever necessary. In this way the patient is kept as free as possible from distressing symptoms.

Total body irradiation is given to patients before they receive a bone marrow or stem (developing) cell transplant for such conditions as leukaemia. The whole body is treated to kill off the cancer cells in the bone marrow as these cells are very sensitive to radiation. The treated marrow is then replaced with new marrow from a donor.

A number of factors are taken into account when planning 'radical' radiotherapy, ie when the treatment is being given in the hope that the cancer will be eradicated:

■ **The type of tumour and how sensitive it is to radiation.** Many lymphomas can be treated successfully because they are easily affected. The liver is rarely treated by radiation because the tumours found here are not very sensitive. Normal liver tissue is easily damaged by radiation so there is the risk that more harm would be done than good.

77

■ **The amount of radiation that would be necessary to achieve a cure.** Some tumour types are much more sensitive to damage by radiation than others.

■ **The site of the tumour.** The prime consideration here is the proximity of the tumour to other vital organs because different organs vary in how sensitive they are to radiation and the dose to these organs needs to be kept to a minimum; the spinal cord is one example.

■ **The size of the tumour.** Large tumours are difficult to control by radiation, and if a large part of the body is treated, side effects from treatment are likely to be more troublesome.

■ **The wishes of the patient.** Irradiating some areas of the body will inevitably cause infertility.

■ **The cosmetic effect.** Sometimes radiation is used to achieve a cure where surgery would be very disfiguring.

■ **The likelihood of cancer elsewhere in the body**. Curative radiotherapy will only work if the cancer is confined to the area treated by the radiotherapy.

How is radiotherapy given?

Radiotherapy treatment is given either externally or internally, depending on the site of the tumour. It is always given at a cancer treatment centre because of the need for specialist equipment. The patient usually attends daily with a break at weekends. Treatment programmes may last up to six weeks depending on the technique used. Because of the tiring regime and daily travel, few patients are able to continue working whilst receiving treatment. If your relative lives a long distance from the hospital it may be less exhausting to arrange accommodation nearby.

External radiation

The treatment plan starts by taking a series of normal x-rays and scans to enable the radiotherapist (the doctor responsible for prescribing the treatment) to obtain an exact picture of the site, size and shape of the tumour. 'Planning' takes place in a simulator, an x-ray machine designed to have the same geometric characteristics as the actual radiotherapy treatment machine. Sometimes the planning involves a 'therapy CT scan' so that the volume of the tumour can be determined with the patient in exactly the same position as they will be when they receive their treatment.

Depending on the complexity of the planning stage the patient may have to visit the simulator several times until the plan is satisfactory. The skin is usually marked with special indelible pens (tiny tattoos) to help the radiographer adjust the treatment machine to deliver the exact dose of radiation. Lasers are used by the radiographers to help with the 'set up'.

For certain areas of the body a plastic shell is made and the marks are placed directly onto this rather than onto the skin. The shell is worn whilst the patient is treated which helps them get into exactly the same position for each session and to keep very still. Plastic shells are commonly used for treating cancers in the head and neck.

The patient lies on a special treatment couch throughout the treatment. The radiographer will 'position' them correctly and set up the radiotherapy machine. The couch may be moved during the process. For some treatment plans there may be several fields to treat so the setting up process is repeated for each area and each treatment lasts for a few minutes only. Radiotherapy is painless. The radiographer operates the machine from outside the room (for their own protection) but a two-way communication system is in place so the patient shouldn't feel too cut off as the radiographer explains exactly what is happening and what to expect. Although the whole process may feel very unfamiliar, the staff will do everything they can to make the visits as stress-free as possible.

Internal radiation

This method involves temporarily inserting a radioactive device into the body and is the method used to treat cancers at sites such as the cervix, uterus (womb) and breast. Until fairly recently it was usual to insert the radioactive source directly into the body, but nowadays it is more usual for an 'after-loading' technique to be used, which avoids exposing the staff involved to radiation. When a cancer of the breast is treated in this way, fine plastic tubes are inserted into the breast whilst the patient is anaesthetised. Radiation physicists calculate how long the radioactive wires will need to stay in place, and these are then threaded through their plastic tubes. Whilst the radioactive implant is in place the patient is nursed in isolation to safeguard other patients and staff. Relatives are asked to stay for only short visits, and particular precautions are needed for pregnant women and children. In some centres the visitors communicate with the patient through a barrier to eliminate the risk. However, once the treatment is over the tubes containing the radioactive wires are taken out, and the patient can safely return home. The staff at the hospital will give patients and relatives clear guidelines about the treatment and what they will be able to do whilst it is taking place.

For treatment to the cervix and womb the radioactive source is placed in the vagina or cavity of the womb. Special applicators are inserted into the area to be treated through the vagina using a remote controlled system. This allows a high dose of radiation to be delivered directly to the area needing the treatment, whilst reducing as far as possible the dose to the uninvolved surrounding tissues. During the treatment the patient is nursed in isolation. Once the treatment is finished the applicators are removed. Radiotherapy treatment using implants or applicators can be uncomfortable.

A different process again is used to treat cancers such as thyroid cancer. These tumours selectively take iodine from the blood, so by giving the person radioactive iodine it is possible to deliver the radioactivity directly into the thyroid cells. Firstly, the cancer and the remainder of the thyroid gland are removed by surgery; secondly, radioactive iodine is injected through a vein. If any residual thyroid tissue or thyroid cancer cells remain they will concentrate the radioactive iodine from the blood and continue to be damaged by the radiation. The patient will be isolated for the duration of the treatment and monitored very closely until the radioactivity has fallen to safe levels as it naturally deteriorates. All stools and urine must be checked until they are clear, and the patient's belongings are scanned with a Geiger counter (see page 254).

The radioactive materials used for internal treatment are chosen for the characteristics of the radiation they emit and their safety. Early treatments used radium but nowadays this has been replaced with safer sources of radioactivity – cobalt, caesium and iridium. The risk to patients, visitors and staff is extremely low; however, very strict rules are always followed when using, moving and disposing of radioactive materials. Any suspected danger of contamination is treated seriously and swiftly. The improvements in the techniques used are among the most beneficial developments that have taken place in recent years.

Side effects

Use of radiation is not totally free of side effects. Clear explanations about what to expect will be given to you and your relative before the treatment starts and there will be opportunities throughout the course of treatment to talk over any problems. The main side effects to be aware of (apart from fatigue) depend on the area being treated. Side effects are divided into those that are immediate, ie that occur during and shortly after treatment, and those which may start months or years after the treatment was given.

Early side effects

- **General tiredness** is typical whatever the type of radiation being given; this is partly due to the treatment and partly due to the demanding regime. Your relative should expect to rest more during the treatment and for a few weeks after it is completed.
- **Redness of the skin** similar to sunburn is usual when the skin itself is being treated or an area close to the surface, particularly under skin folds. Any soreness will heal quickly once treatment stops. The staff at the centre will offer advice on skin care and the use of body lotions and talcum powder.
- **Hair loss** only happens if hair-bearing skin has been irradiated: the scalp, beard area, armpits or pubic area. The hair will usually grow again, but this depends on the dose of radiation that has been given. If bald patches remain, wigs are available

for temporary or permanent cover in the same way as for chemotherapy patients. (For tips on hair care, see page 108.)

■ **Difficulty in swallowing with a sore, dry mouth** is common during treatment to the head and neck, and a sore throat is usual if the oesophagus is treated. Certain infections, such as thrush, are common and may need treatment with anti-fungal therapy. Loss of taste may persist for a while. Pay careful attention to dental hygiene, use a mouth wash and take pain killers and avoid spicy foods and alcohol if the discomfort is too great.

■ **Diarrhoea, nausea and occasional vomiting** can occur when the abdominal and pelvic areas are treated. Anti-sickness and anti-diarrhoea medicines help enormously and additional nourishing drinks prevent weight loss.

■ **Cystitis,** causing frequency and burning when passing urine, may follow treatment to the bladder. The problem is short lived and can be treated with medication to increase the alkalinity of the urine.

■ **Somnolence or the 'sleepy syndrome'** occurs about four to six weeks after radiotherapy to the brain; your relative may become very sleepy and have no energy for a week or two having had no problems when the treatment finished. Somnolence settles without treatment.

Later side effects

■ **Skin changes** are rare with modern radiotherapy techniques, but if the skin itself has been treated then the affected area will become paler and the skin thinner; sometimes little blood vessels show through.

■ **Lymphoedema** may occur if surgery to lymph nodes is followed by radiotherapy (see page 105).

■ **Shortness of breath** may occur a few months after a course of radiotherapy, and usually improves after a few weeks or with a short course of steroids. Occasionally it remains as a problem.

■ **Loss of fertility and an early menopause** are unavoidable for younger women who receive radiation to the ovaries. Hormone replacement therapy can be given to patients if menopausal symptoms are severe, and counselling will always be offered for those people who are distressed at the thought of being sterile.

■ **Loss of fertility for men** may be avoided if one testicle only is being treated; if both testicles are affected, the option of storing sperm is available. Radiotherapy to the pelvic area has no direct affect on sexual function.

■ **Narrowing of the vagina** can cause discomfort after radioactive implants. Use of lubricants and regular dilation of the vagina can help to overcome the problem.

Hygiene

Fiona, cancer centre nurse

'There are many myths about whether or not it is possible to wash the area whilst the course of treatment is in progress. It is usually quite OK to gently wash the affected area and to take normal baths or showers; rest assured, gentle hygiene to the area will not do any harm and the radiographers looking after your relative will give clear instructions about what they may or must not do. Feeling fresh and clean makes people feel better so do offer help to your relative if they don't feel up to taking full care of themselves.'

The restrictions of radiotherapy

All courses of radiotherapy are planned taking into account the health of the person, the type and extent of the tumour and the effects of radiation on other nearby tissue. Due thought (and explanation) will always be given to what will happen in the future if the cancer recurs. Unfortunately, there is a maximum dose of radiation that can be given to any site and this may mean that it is not possible to re-treat this area with radiation if the cancer returns. Certain tissues, such as the brain, the spinal cord and the liver can only be treated with relatively low doses of radiation if over-dosing is to be avoided. In particular, the bone marrow is affected by radiotherapy and chemotherapy which results in failure of the bone marrow to produce all types of blood cells, and a lowering of the level of these cells in the blood. If, for any of these reasons, it is not possible for your relative to have a further course of radiotherapy, he or she will need support. Do be sure that they understand the reasons why, and what alternative care is possible.

Hormone treatment

Hormone therapy relies on the effects of substances produced by endocrine glands (chemical messengers) to help slow down the growth of the cancer. The output of hormones from certain glands (the pituitary, the thyroid, the adrenals, the ovaries and the testes) directly control the growth of some tissues; for example, there is a direct link between the sex hormone oestrogen produced by the ovaries and the growth of breast tissue. Towards the end of the nineteenth century a surgeon discovered that removing the ovaries of women with advanced breast cancer had an immediate effect on the progression of the disease. Although this halt was only temporary the research that followed showed that manipulation of blood hormone levels can affect the growth of certain cancers. Hormone therapy is used mainly to treat cancer of the breast, the uterus, the ovaries and the prostate gland.

There are two main ways that the activity of hormone-producing glands can be altered. The production of the hormone can be stopped – by removal of the gland, by radiation or by suppressing the gland's action. Removal of the testicles (castration) was a significant treatment for prostate cancer for many years although it has been largely superseded by other methods. Alternatively, the action of the hormone can be reduced or blocked. The best example here is the use of the drug Tamoxifen in treating breast cancer; it blocks the action of oestrogen within the cell, discouraging cell growth.

Hormone treatment is generally very safe with few side effects. The choice of hormone therapy will depend on the type of tumour involved and the probability that it will respond to treatment. For example, although some breast cancers respond very well to a hormone treatment such as tamoxifen, others do not. Although hormone treatments are generally safe they are not without any side effects; for example, there is a slight rise in the number of cardiovascular (heart-related) problems in men who may be treated with oestrogen, and so oestrogen therapy would not be recommended for men with an existing heart problem.

Immunotherapy

The concept of immunotherapy is not new. Attempts at finding suitable agents that might immunise the body against cancer have been the basis for experiments since the same principles were first recognised for impeding infectious diseases. However, trials that injected animals with cancer tissue in order to produce cancer antibodies that would stimulate the immune systems have never developed beyond the experimental stages.

More recent scientific research is looking at methods in which drugs can be used to change the way the body behaves, a so-called 'biological response'. The most widely used substance that achieves this effect is interferon, a substance that occurs naturally in the body. Immunotherapy is used alongside other drug therapy to stimulate the body's immune system. Certain lymphomas and widespread cancers of the kidney are offered treatment in this way.

Following treatment

After the chosen course of treatment is over, your relative will be given a follow-up date to see the specialist again. The length of time between completion of the therapy or operation and the timing of the appointment may depend on your relative's state of health and the length of waiting list at the outpatient clinic. If you are concerned about any aspect of the illness in the meantime, or your relative's condition changes, the GP is always available as the first point of call.

He or she will have been fully informed by the hospital of your relative's progress. Your relative may already have met a specialist nurse during their treatment who will also be able to give advice or help.

Going to work

It is unlikely that many patients would wish to continue working while receiving treatment because of the effort needed to undergo therapy, although some people can and do manage to carry on working through treatment. If your relative does continue working, tell the cancer team so that treatment schedules can fit around their work. Employed people suffering from cancer are given rights under legislation that protect against discrimination. People are entitled to ask for their job to be kept open (although the provision may depend on their individual contract) and to expect that their employer makes reasonable allowances for their illness when they return to work; employees do not have to inform their employer of the nature of their illness if they do not wish, although if there is an occupational health scheme in place the occupational health doctor or nurse will be able to assess if the person is fit to continue with their work. If a person is dismissed on health grounds they have the right to challenge the action depending on the length of their employment. Independent advice can be obtained from a Citizens Advice Bureau (see telephone directory for contact details) or a solicitor.

Unorthodox treatments

The conventional treatments described above are relatively well known. Some patients also seek out other less well documented therapies, especially when they feel that established treatments have failed. It must be stressed, however, that the examples of alternative treatments described below are not 'miracle cures'. Occasionally accounts of spectacular results are reported in the press or promotional books written by practitioners. Unfortunately,

despite these public claims there are no proven cures and scientif-
ically-controlled trials have so far failed to achieve the same results
in other patients.

Generally, complementary therapies are used alongside conventional therapy. There is no reason why you and your relative should
not find out about, or use, complementary therapies alongside
orthodox treatments if you so wish. Sometimes such therapies can
bring relief during stressful times for you and your relative; many
complementary therapies have been practised for centuries bringing emotional and physical relief. Reputable therapists never make
direct claims that their methods will cure a disease; instead they
will support the view that natural therapies may help to promote
healing. The important advice is to use the therapies sensibly and
to work with the orthodox cancer team.

The non-traditional treatments listed below are given as examples
only and do not cover the full range of therapies. This topic is covered in more detail in Chapter 7, with descriptions of complementary
therapies that can be of benefit to you and your relative.

Complementary therapies

- **Acupressure** is an ancient skill practised in China and Japan
  for over 3,000 years. It combines massage with acupuncture
  principles and is thought to have been the forerunner of
  acupuncture. It does not use needles. Acupressure is believed
  to improve the body's healing powers, prevent illness and promote energy. Practitioners work on known pressure points
  with thumbs, finger tips, etc, to balance the flow of energy
  called Qi, which runs throughout the body via meridians or
  invisible channels. Acupressure relieves the symptoms of many
  conditions and is best used in conjunction with other natural or
  orthodox treatments.
- **Aromatherapy** combines the restorative properties of aromatic plant essences with the soothing effects of gentle
  massage (see page 243). This therapy is a good one to try if
  complementary treatments are new to you.

- **Faith healing** is based on the belief that positive or 'right' thinking can cure or relieve illness. The belief is particularly strong when practised within a religious setting where healing through spiritual means is preached. Patients are attended by non-medical healers who believe that faith healing enhances the body's natural defences by reducing the effects of stress. It can reinforce the mental attitude of patients so that they feel better even though their condition may not be improved.
- **Homeopathy** relies on the principle of treating like with like, whereby minute quantities of a natural substance are given to stimulate the body's own healing power (see page 247).
- **Reflexology** involves massaging areas of the body (mainly the feet) which practitioners believe helps to free blockages in energy pathways (see page 249).

Alternative therapies

- **Naturopathy** is an approach to 'natural healing' where no drugs (or radiotherapy) are used and the belief in cures is based on special diets, exercise and practical therapies. Naturopathy concentrates on helping the body to cure itself. Like faith healing it encourages people to think positively about their problem and not to concentrate on the negative aspects of the illness. Practitioners attempt to identify the underlying cause of the illness and to treat this rather than deal with the symptoms. Each person is treated as an individual and the therapist takes an holistic (whole body) approach. They seek to complement and support traditional medicine.
- **Bristol Cancer Help Centre** opened in 1980 with a clear vision to provide a new, holistic approach for cancer patients that offers a link between orthodox medicine and the complementary therapies and care. The 'approach' promoted by the Centre uses a combination of therapies and self-help techniques focusing on the patient's emotional and spiritual health and state of mind. The therapy works alongside medical treatment to confront fears and teaches that the patient has control over many of the important factors that affect health.

The Centre staff believe that people who react with a positive approach to the diagnosis of cancer are more able to help themselves. For example, the Centre teaches that patients can strengthen their immune system and thus enhance their potential for recovery.

The Bristol Cancer Help Centre therapy programme comprises a starter pack, an introductory course, a residential course, follow-up days and telephone support. It must be noted that the approach promoted by the Centre is an alternative form of therapy that should complement, not replace, orthodox treatment. Many patients who have used the services of the Centre find the facilities and self-help elements very supportive.

For more *i*nformation

The following national charities all offer materials and advice covering most aspects of cancer treatments and care. Many charities also undertake and/or support research into cancer. For details of how to contact these organisations and other specific cancer-related charities, see the 'Useful addresses' section starting on page 258; the names of the organisations are presented in alphabetical order.

- ***i*** **Bristol Cancer Help Centre** offers a range of services for patients and their supporters including a therapy programme, education and research and a retail shop.

- ***i*** **CancerBACUP** (British Association of Cancer United Patients and their families and friends) offers a range of services including advice, information and a telephone helpline.

- ***i*** **Cancer Research UK** promotes research into causes, symptoms and treatment and provides publications and information about cancer.

- ***i*** **Macmillan Cancer Relief** offers a range of services, including specialist cancer nurses, palliative care specialist nurses (often referred to as 'Macmillan' nurses), pain relief, emotional support, grants and education.

- ***i*** **Marie Curie Cancer Care** provides a range of services including education and training for health professionals, nursing care at home and specialist palliative care in centres throughout the country.

ⓘ **National Cancer Alliance** is a voluntary group of patients and health-care professionals formed to improve cancer services and voice concerns and opinions of people affected by cancer. It offers a range of services, including advice and information.

ⓘ **Sue Ryder Care** provides specialist palliative care services at seven homes in the UK.

Conclusion

This chapter has given basic information about the most common tests and treatments for cancer. Tests are a necessary part of the diagnostic process as most treatments cannot be started until the doctor has a clear picture of the nature and extent of the illness. Understanding why tests are necessary often helps patients to get through a frightening and unpleasant experience, particularly when they are already feeling unwell. As a carer you may be the person who accompanies your relative to the clinic so it is vital that you also understand what is happening, to boost your confidence and improve the quality of care that you provide. Most people in this situation feel apprehensive – you are not alone if you find these visits daunting. A quick glance around the waiting room will show a row of anxious faces. Remember that it is all right to ask questions about any aspect of your relative's illness or care that you do not understand. Try to remain positive (and realistic), as a resolute outlook gives hope and hope brings courage. Future chapters discuss how you and your relative can deal with some of the practical issues and help manage the inevitable stress.

3 Wellbeing

The chances are that as you read this chapter your relative is already past the stages outlined in the previous chapters, has completed the necessary tests and is receiving treatments or, better still, they are beginning to recover and picking up the threads of life again. This chapter offers information and advice to help you move forward. Hopefully, you are all feeling relieved that the treatment phase is over, with its associated fatigue, side effects and anxiety, and are looking at the next period with optimism; your relative endured the trauma of the therapies but no doubt you and other family and friends suffered along with them while offering care and support.

Whatever the outcome of tests and treatments, there is still plenty that your relative can do to build up strength to deal with their situation. Changes can be made to lifestyle that will reduce the future risks and help your relative adapt to new circumstances. For example:

■ Managing and improving diet to boost energy and organising eating habits after a colostomy or removal of the stomach.

■ Learning to live with changes in body shape or function such as stoma care or a breast prosthesis.

■ Giving up smoking – it's still a good idea to give up, even if smoking was not a contributing factor.

- *Taking appropriate exercise to increase fitness and keep the heart healthy.*

- *Managing sexual relationships, if this is a part of your relative's life.*

- *Chapter 8 offers a range of methods to manage stress and cope with pressure during this anxious time.*

The thought of making major lifestyle changes on top of everything else that has happened may be daunting, so the chapter starts by offering some tips about making changes in general. Not all the advice here will apply to the person you care for, so pick out the information that is relevant.

Jean

'I can cope better if I am busy so I felt less frustrated when the doctor gave me a list of things to go away and do. I sent away for information and made some immediate changes to our diet.'

Mark, a GP

'I always reassure my patients and their relatives that there is much they can do to help themselves. I find relatives always adjust better if they are allowed to take an active part in the care and treatment, however small.'

Any operation or treatment for cancer is serious and you are probably fearful that the cancer might recur again quickly, whatever the oncologist might have said. It takes time to come to terms with what has happened and to believe that there is a future. Many people feel anxious during the convalescent stage and need reassurance that life can resume again. A great deal of support will be available in the early days to help you all begin the process of getting back to normal. Looking after someone who is ill brings responsibilities and you will want to do your best for them in every possible way. Talk to your doctor or nurse, follow their advice and you and your relative will soon slip into a new pattern of life.

Fact box

Here are a few positive facts to help you and your relative overcome any anxieties:

- Many people make an excellent recovery after cancer treatment.
- Most parts of the body are designed for self-repair so will heal well after surgery.
- Many body organs function adequately when damaged or reduced in size and can easily compensate for any lowered capacity.
- After surgery or other therapies it's normal to tire more easily and not a sign of problems.
- Self-help is a great boost to recovery.

Making changes

A change in circumstances is always triggered by some event, however insignificant. If you think about major changes in the past, something happened that set you off on a new course of action. Sometimes the event is not within your control and you feel unsettled until you have come to terms with the new situation. The process is easier to deal with if you allow time to work your way naturally through a series of stages.

The first period is often called the *'unfreezing' stage*. It's the time to let everything settle down and accept that you can't put the clock back. The illness of your relative is the event that triggered the change. It's important that you both spend time talking about how this situation has affected your lives; think about the past; let relatives and friends offer support and don't try to block out any emotional feelings because you won't be able to plan for the future whilst you still feel upset about what has happened. Give yourself permission to grieve about the past, it's quite normal to want to do this when a traumatic event has occurred.

The next stage is called *'moving forward'*. It's the time to start putting changes into action. Your relative may be on the road to recovery or entering a stable phase and you will both feel ready to make plans for the future. Don't rush this stage and talk to other people if you feel anxious about making decisions. Your plans might centre on a range of issues covering financial arrangements, short and long term health, living accommodation and other practical matters. They all need careful thought.

When you and your relative have made decisions and begun to sort out the immediate issues, you are entering stage three. This time is called the *'re-freezing'* period and it only becomes *solid* when you both feel comfortable about the changes that have taken place. This final stage won't happen swiftly, so don't be alarmed if it takes a while before life feels close to normal again. Be honest with yourselves about accepting the changes because pretending and putting on a brave face when you feel anxious inside is also stressful.

Jane

'I will always remember the chemotherapy nurse saying to me, "Understanding makes coping easier." She was right.'

If you or your relative are having difficulty accepting that change is taking place, it might help to talk about what is holding you up. Sometimes problems are perceived by the mind to be greater than they are in reality. It's better if you can face a problem squarely, otherwise you may think that you have dealt with it but, rather than resolving the 'worry', it springs up again in another guise. This may be because you haven't truly come to terms with the problem, so it continues to dominate your thoughts. The change process is a slow business so don't dash into a false sense of acceptance. As you sort out problems, bit by bit, the nightmare of dealing with the huge change will feel less of a burden.

In a quiet moment think about this list.

- **Do** look forward.
- **Do** make a list of the good things in life, however trivial.
- **Do** talk to someone about difficult decisions.
- **Do** accept that life moves forward.
- **Do** acknowledge your own feelings.
- **Do** try to find someone to talk through your feelings with if you need to.
- **Do** remember help is available.

- **Don't** rush yourselves.
- **Don't** bottle up feelings.
- **Don't** feel guilty.
- **Don't** try to place blame.
- **Don't** look over your shoulder hankering for a 'better' past.

Adjusting to change

Sylvia and Derek

'After the shock of the cancer the clinic nurse gave us some advice – move forward gently, as time passes the blow lessens and you learn to adapt.'

Few issues can be more frightening than the thought of living with a body that has fundamentally changed. Altered body image and reduced function need to be accepted and managed and this may take a great deal of time and patience for you and your relative.

The creation of a colostomy or ileostomy and the removal of one or both breasts (mastectomy) are common examples of body-altering surgery emphasised in this chapter and problems such as hair loss are covered. However, there are many other ways that a body can be disfigured or its power reduced. Hospital staff will offer sensitive advice and be very supportive whatever the cause and will understand that any type of change may give rise to worry and emotional distress. The specialist nurses are highly trained and will have helped many other patients adapt to the process of change.

Reconstructive and plastic surgery techniques, if appropriate, are readily available for cancer patients and it is quite amazing what can be achieved, whether the affected body part is visible or not. External wounds in prominent areas can be disguised by plastic (cosmetic) surgery, limb shapes can be conserved and internal organs reconstructed. The extent to which these techniques can be applied depend very much on the nature of the cancer and its treatment. Expert advice will be offered to help your relative make important decisions about whether or not to go ahead. A course of plastic surgery may be long and arduous so if your relative does not wish to proceed it is important that their decision is accepted and supported. People who decline further operations often feel they are being cowardly if they say 'no', or they may continue to endure treatment to please others.

Stoma care

Colostomy

Fewer people now leave hospital with a permanent colostomy than in the past. When a section of bowel is removed from the intestine the surgeon will aim to join the two ends of healthy tissue together. If this is not possible, a false opening (stoma) is made onto the outside of the abdominal wall to allow the passage of faeces (stools). The protruding piece of bowel is sewn to the surface skin forming a colostomy (large intestine) or ileostomy (small intestine). Many stomas are created as temporary measures only, to give the intestine below the surgical site time to heal, and closed at a later date. A permanent colostomy is usually necessary only if the tumour was removed from the lower part of the rectum where extensive surgery is necessary to remove the tumour completely.

The word stoma comes from a Greek word meaning 'mouth' or 'opening', ie colostomy means 'opening in the colon'. The stoma looks like a small, puckered mouth-shaped opening. It is dark pink in colour and is without feeling, despite it's raw appearance. The siting of the opening depends largely on where the section of bowel is removed. Patients are encouraged to think beforehand how the position could affect their future activities, posture and clothing style. It is also important to be able to see it clearly to make bag changing easy. A stoma nurse always advises where to mark the site.

After food has been digested in the normal way, the waste matter (indigestible fibre and water) collects in the colon. When the waste material reaches the opening the stools are passed into a disposable bag attached to the skin with an adhesive rim. The bags are removed and emptied or destroyed as necessary. Whether a temporary or permanent stoma has been created, the procedure is the same. A range of bag designs is available in terms of size, fixing style, materials and emptying arrangements, and your stoma therapist will be able to help your relative find what will suit them best.

At first the waste matter is ejected randomly as it arrives at the stoma, but colostomy owners usually find that a regular pattern develops in much the same way as before. Stools that are passed through a stoma may be less formed than motions that would normally stay longer in the bowel, especially if the stoma is situated high up in the colon, but users need not be concerned, colostomy bags are strong and well designed for their purpose.

It takes a while to feel comfortable about dealing with a colostomy and adjusting to the changes in body appearance but every foreseeable aspect of living with a stoma is covered before leaving the ward. Permanent colostomy bag users soon enjoy a normal attitude towards life with almost total freedom of lifestyle, including sexual activity (see page 125). Some people, who adopt the habit of flushing out their colostomy at a regular time each day, find they can reduce the times when they need to use a bag and after a while many people get to know which foods to avoid and which foods add bulk to the stool.

Ileostomy

The guidelines for dealing with an ileostomy are similar to those given above for a colostomy. The surgery technique used to create the opening is the same as a colostomy except that the stoma is created in the ileum (small intestine) rather than the colon. Waste matter arriving at the site of an ileostomy has travelled a shorter distance through the bowel than material that exits via the colon, therefore less water has been absorbed from the faeces. The waste matter leaving the body through an iloestomy is usually more liquid and in greater quantities than from a colostomy. A person with an ileostomy (ileostomist) needs to wear a drainable pouch so that it may be emptied regularly – usually several times a day.

What support can your relative expect to receive?

■ Information and advice from a specially trained stoma therapist, a specialist nurse who will offer practical help and advice and psychological support. Care at home is available from the stoma therapist, and from community nurses.

■ Regular stoma clinics are provided by many hospitals.

■ A free prescription service for all stoma supplies available from GPs, if the colostomy is permanent. The prescription can be dispensed in the usual way at a local pharmacy or through a specialist supplier.

■ A dietitian can offer advice if dietary problems occur and your relative finds it difficult to achieve regular motions with formed stools.

■ Support from specialist organisations (see page 102).

■ Details about how to make contact with other colostomists and ileostomists who will offer support.

Everyday activities

Once your relative has recovered from the ordeal of the surgery, they will want to settle back into a normal routine as quickly as possible. Offer lots of support including reassurance and practical, hands-on help. However proficient they become eventually at bag changing and dealing with post-colostomy life, the early days may bring a few problems. Self-help is always a good start when dealing with minor worries but remember the stoma care nurse is available if problems persist.

As your relative starts to pick up the threads of life, it may be reassuring if a close friend or relative offers to accompany them when they first go out in case they need assistance. Do a bit of discreet research beforehand about facilities at local venues to avoid embarrassment. Check out toilet facilities and whether there is a private area to attend to a stoma. Space is important as it could be difficult to manoeuvre in cramped conditions.

Wind and odour

In reality the apprehension may prove to be worse than the actuality. Excessive wind can be a regular problem for some people but it's more likely to be the result of eating particular foods. Certain foods such as onions, beans and carbonated drinks are well known wind generators. The solution is no different than for anyone else – learn what to avoid or live with the consequences! There should be no need to change to a special diet.

Sue

'My husband developed really bad wind when he first came home from hospital. We soon got over the embarrassment and had a few good family laughs. Seeing the funny side did us the world of good and helped us to support each other.'

Odour escaping from the bag is almost impossible as many pouches have a built-in filter that allows gas to disperse and absorbs unpleasant smells. Modern bags have an odour-proof lining. Deodorant sprays are available for use when changing pouches if your relative is concerned about disagreeable smells.

Tips to help avoid wind

■ Chew food slowly and thoroughly.
■ Try to prevent swallowing air while eating – eat with mouth closed, don't talk and chew at the same time and don't gulp down large amounts of fluid.
■ Don't over-eat or miss out on meals – small, routine meals help to regulate digestion.
■ Keep a food diary to identify foods that cause problems and experiment for a while – it may be the combination of several foods that create wind or it may be the time of day the meal is eaten.
■ If wind is worse at night causing sleep problems, try taking the main meal at midday.
■ Don't be shy about leaving unwanted food on the plate when eating out – unless other people know about the colostomy there is no need to explain or apologise.

Diarrhoea

Loose stools can be distressing and uncomfortable for anyone and the causes and solutions are much the same for all sufferers. The main culprits are: tummy bugs, unsuitable food, excessive fluid, anxiety and stress. If the problem is temporary stay close to a toilet or suitable changing facility. If the diarrhoea recurs or doesn't ease up it's important to seek advice: identify the problem food if possible and exclude it from the menu for a while or discuss the problem with your GP or nurse.

Constipation

Similar advice applies to constipation, ie if the problem continues it may be necessary to talk to a dietitian or stoma care nurse. Firstly, check out whether diet is causing the problem as certain foods such as eggs, rice and too much fibre can make the stools very firm. By way of a solution try increasing (slightly) the foods that tend to have a loosening effect and drink more fluid. Whatever your relative tries, suggest that they do it in moderation as it's important to achieve a balance and not swing between the two extremes.

Alcohol

It's quite OK for stoma owners to drink any alcohol they enjoy. Consume in moderation is the best advice, although too much beer or lager may lead to excess wind and diarrhoea.

Jim

'My brother loves a pint and was unsure about how much alcohol to drink. The lads in the pub knew about his cancer and I asked them on the quiet not to pressure him into overdoing the rounds.'

Holidays and recreation

Encourage your relative to continue doing whatever they feel comfortable to achieve. A colostomy should make little difference to travel arrangements or leisure activities but a few precautions would be advisable. For example, carry a stoma care pack to facilitate easy pouch changing (tissues, spray, etc); keep this accessible at all times to avoid undue worry, especially during air travel when passengers and their main luggage are separated; check out facilities beforehand, particularly if it's long distance (many tourist offices in larger towns keep details of public toilet facilities and most department stores have toilets); contact coach operators to ensure that toilets will be available on board (if not, ask for the expected length of the journey and add a bit for traffic delays); take a good supply of anti-diarrhoea medication in case of problems and, finally, check travel insurance policies well in advance in case there are clauses that need clarification.

101

For more *i*nformation

ⓘ The British Colostomy Association offers help, information and advice to all stoma patients and their carers (address on page 260). A range of free leaflets is available on request.

ⓘ CancerBACUP booklet *Understanding cancer of the colon* (address on page 261).

ⓘ Ileostomy and Internal Pouch Support Group (address on page 266).

Breast reconstruction

Great advances have been made in the field of breast surgery; however, for some cases (male and female) the most appropriate treatment remains a mastectomy. Such a decision would be made where the cancer is close to, or includes the nipple, or where a large tumour is present in a person with a small breast.

Post-operative choices and techniques

All units carrying out breast surgery should have a breast care specialist nurse attached. This specialist nurse is able to advise on all aspects of breast care from diagnosis, through surgery and treatment, to advice on post-operative treatment and care, including the use of bras and prostheses.

Breast prosthesis

Following a mastectomy your relative will be offered a prosthesis, an artificial breast worn inside the bra. Prostheses are made of soft silicone in a range of sizes, shapes and colours, to achieve as natural a look as possible. Immediately after the operation your relative may be given a soft, light fabric prosthesis to wear until her chest wall has healed completely. Women who wish to augment a small breast reconstruction can use a partial prosthesis. The structure allows the prosthesis to fit neatly and safely into a bra, with a nipple outline to give a well-balanced appearance.

> *Freda*
>
> 'When the breast care nurse told us about care of prostheses she put my mother in touch with a support group and she spoke to other women who had undergone a similar experience.'

Methods and timing

Reconstruction of a breast(s) may be performed after a mastectomy or lumpectomy to restore the breast to a size and shape that is similar to the original. Several methods are used according to which technique (or combination of techniques) best suits the area on which the surgeon must work, and taking into account the wishes of the patient. Much help and advice will be offered by the cancer team before and after the operation.

The timing of the reconstruction also depends on several factors; for example, some surgeons prefer to do all the surgery at one time, whereas others recommend a time gap to allow the operation site to recover; radiotherapy and chemotherapy usually mean a delay of several months. Your relative's views will always be sought and at this emotional time she may need extra support and the chance to talk over the options. The waiting lists for breast reconstruction surgery are quite long in some areas.

The idea of a breast reconstruction is attractive for many women, particularly if they are very concerned by the thought of a traumatic change in body shape or by the bother of dealing with a separate prosthesis (artificial replacement). The psychological and practical advantages of a permanent reconstruction outweigh the disadvantages because dressing is easier and body image more acceptable. However, it is important to understand that the new breast will not be identical to the one removed during surgery – the new tissue will be less sensitive and the reconstructed shape of the flesh and nipple will look different. Once your relative is fully dressed the appearance is very agreeable, with little outward sign that the two breasts differ.

Occasionally cosmetic surgery work is performed on the healthy breast to make it easier for the surgeon to match the new reconstruction; for example, the existing breast may be reduced in size or lifted. Additional surgery for cosmetic effect would only be done after discussion about the advantages and disadvantages for your relative.

Reconstruction techniques

There are two main types of reconstruction performed in the UK using implanted, artificial material or a tissue flap using transplanted tissue taken from elsewhere in the body.

An artificial implant uses either saline (salt) fluid or silicone gel inserted into the body within a textured, silicone casing. The saline fluid is a natural substance, so it is less likely to cause problems if it seeps out, but a saline-type implant feels less realistic than a silicone model. Encapsulated silicone gel implants have been used for many years and there is little risk associated with this type of procedure. The main problems highlighted in the media have been linked to use of silicone injections where a compound was injected directly into breast tissue. Reports of leakage and infection caused women to be fearful of the technique, with claims of autoimmune disorders developing. The use of silicone injections is now banned in the UK and the USA and monitoring of all silicone implants is undertaken regularly by the Department of Health. Following a review in 1998 the report found that 'there is no good evidence of an abnormal immune response ... and there is no reason to stop using silicone implants' (CancerBACUP).

After-care

Immediately after the surgery the area will be taken care of by nursing staff, who will advise on personal hygiene. For example, showers are better than baths and careful drying of the area is important. Many doctors advise gently massaging the area daily with oils or creams to keep the skin soft and elastic, and to help reduce the amount of fibrous tissue that can form around the capsule.

A support bra worn during the day and at night time is suggested by some surgeons to help reduce the dragging, whereas another school of thought recommends wearing a normal bra or none at all to encourage the new breast to develop its own natural shape. Your relative must be guided by her own surgeon. Full movement is usually recovered after about six weeks. A physiotherapist will teach suitable arm exercises to aid mobility. It is important to continue to observe the reconstructed breast regularly for signs of change and the breast care nurse will tell your relative what to look out for.

For more *i*nformation

i Breast Cancer Care offer a range of breast care and post-mastectomy leaflets (address on page 259).

i CancerBACUP booklet *Understanding breast reconstruction* (address on page 261).

Lymphoedema

Lymphoedema is a build up of lymphatic fluid in the tissue that lies directly under the surface of the skin. It collects in the space between cells and can produce swelling which causes discomfort and loss of mobility. The condition develops because the lymphatic system fails to drain the fluid adequately and return it to the circulation. This problem may occur following damage after surgery or radiation. Lymphoedema of the arm following treatment for breast cancer is not uncommon, especially if some or all of the lymph nodes in the armpit area have been removed or the armpit area has been treated by radiotherapy. It may also affect the lower limbs after treatment involving the pelvic or groin lymph nodes; sometimes this can be a symptom that the cancer is progressing in the pelvis.

Lymphoedema cannot be cured but the symptoms can be kept well under control. Early treatment is advisable as it brings better results. The treatment will help to manage the pain, reduce limb size and increase movement. The patient and their relatives are given advice on skin care and taught special exercises and massage to assist the lymph drainage. For mild or moderate lymphoedema, a special support sleeve can be fitted. If the problem is severe a technique for bandaging the arm with a multi-layered bandage can be applied over a number of days to reduce the swelling and when the lymphoedema has improved sufficiently, support hosiery is fitted to maintain the improvement. Your relative will receive advice on lymphoedema either from a breast care specialist nurse or be referred to a specialist lymphoedema clinic.

Head and neck surgery

Body image is especially important when the area is always visible. Disfigurement of the head or neck can be disguised if the person so wishes with carefully placed accessories but it is almost impossible to completely hide or disguise scarring on the face. Plastic surgery is now a common technique, particularly in the field of cosmetic surgery, and the results can be very pleasing.

Nicki, cancer centre nurse

'Help your relative to draw the eye away from scar tissue by paying close attention to other aspects of their dress and making the most of special features. Make-up and jewellery for women and smart ties and sweaters for men are easy ways to look good and boost self-confidence. Perhaps some lessons from a trained beautician could be arranged to help someone apply their make-up to the best advantage. As time passes, hopefully your relative will feel less conspicuous and realise that people generally pay scant attention to facial disfigurements.'

Hair care and permanent hair loss

'Will I lose my hair?' is an anxious question asked by many cancer patients when they are first told about proposed chemotherapy or radiotherapy. The reasons why hair drops out are given more fully in Chapter 2 (see pages 71 and 81), together with basic tips to help cope with a temporary loss. This section offers advice and information about hair care for longer-term hair loss.

Hair loss after chemotherapy is rarely permanent as the hair-producing cells begin to recover even before the course of treatment is over. The new hair may be different in appearance with changes in colour, texture and initial curliness. After about six months hair growth settles down with little difference to original hair.

Hair re-growth after radiotherapy may also be good, although recovery time is longer – from six to twelve months after treatment ends. Unfortunately, permanent hair loss does affect some patients after radiotherapy with little or no hair regenerating. The extent to which hair loss is likely to be permanent depends on the dose of radiotherapy given to the hair-bearing skin. The radiotherapist will be able to give a more accurate opinion based on your relative's individual case.

Molly, cancer centre nurse

'Loss of hair, whether temporary or permanent, frequently gives rise to powerful emotions for patients and their relatives – perhaps because the change in appearance is so obvious and it serves as a constant reference to the illness. Your relative may wish to talk about their looks but may be unsure about your reaction. You could set the ball rolling by saying that, although you feel upset on their behalf, you are not appalled by the lack of hair. Give them time to open up and then share feelings with each other – be ready for expressions of anger and despair. Cancer specialist nurses can arrange for either of you to talk to a counsellor or put new patients in touch with other cancer patients with similar disabilities.'

Tips on hair care

- Ask your relative if they would like help with hair care; it will show that you are not bothered by the look or feel of their bare scalp if you wash and dry their hair for them.
- Hair loss often happens quite quickly after treatment begins, so dispose of fallen hair discreetly and gently remove stray locks from their back and shoulders. A hair net or soft hat collects loose hair at night and helps keep the scalp warm.
- Provide a selection of fashionable hats and scarves for your relative to wear temporarily, that match their clothes and complexion.
- When new growth begins, or if some residual hair is present, suggest a short haircut in an attractive head-hugging style. A short style is good for two reasons – it prevents too much weight dragging on the damaged roots and gives the appearance of a uniform length until a thicker growth is established.
- Many hairdressers are willing to make home visits for cancer patients and some hospitals have hairdressing salons.
- Buy a soft brush suitable for a baby if existing combs and brushes are heavy and sharp.
- Offer to nourish the scalp by massaging with appropriate hair products and use only mild shampoo.
- Dry hair by towelling gently rather than using a drier as heat can make the hair brittle.
- Suggest that your relative allows their hair to hang naturally as it grows rather than holding it back with bands or clips.
- Avoid using strong chemicals that could damage the new growth for several months after treatment ends.
- Remind your relative that the chemicals in deodorants could cause irritation if they have lost under-arm hair. Light talcum powder will help absorb moisture and give a pleasant smell. If the armpit area has been treated by radiotherapy the sweat glands stop functioning so anti-perspirants are not needed.

Long-term solutions

Wigs and hairpieces are the most common ways of covering up permanent hair loss and there are practical ways to protect a temporary bare or patchy scalp, such as hats, scarves and turbans. If your relative wishes to seek an independent source, ask at local hair salons or larger department stores. VAT is not chargeable for cancer patients but the appropriate forms must be completed at the time of purchase as a claim cannot be made later. Free wigs are available under the Benefits Agency (DWP) provision for hospital inpatients and people (or their partners) who receive certain benefits (see leaflet WF11 from your local Benefit Agency office). Subsidised rates are offered through the NHS and grants are obtainable from some cancer charities for people who do not qualify for free wigs. Advice and information is readily available. Ask for details at the cancer centre, from a GP surgery or social worker or contact one of the cancer helplines on pages 258–274 for a list of wig suppliers.

Wigs are made from synthetic materials or real hair; there are advantages and disadvantages to both types. For example, cost, ease of care and weight are better with artificial fibre wigs but natural hair looks more realistic and lasts longer. Real hair wigs are not usually available under the NHS.

Achieving a secure fit is very important. Suggest that your relative bends over and shakes their head to check for slippage and ask about methods of attaching wigs, such as double-sided tape. Some wigs adjust to head size. If your relative's scalp feels sensitive when the wig is in place, ask about hypo-allergic linings and fixing tape or cotton skull caps. Wig after-care is important so make sure the manufacturer provides clear information and ask the local salon for help. Synthetic materials can be washed and dried at home easily but real hair usually requires professional cleaning. Hairdressers are often trained in wig care and many would be able to re-style a wig if fashions change or your relative fancies a new look.

For more *i*nformation

i CancerBACUP booklet *Coping with hair loss* (address on page 261).

General health care

Although many aspects of health – family history and previous exposure to carcinogens – are fixed, it's never too late to make changes for the better or to make the best of present health. Taking a look at everyday lifestyle is the easiest starting place.

Diet

Georgina, a dietitian

'The word "diet" usually conjures up images of sparse portions and grumbling hunger pangs; however, in this context "diet" means "what your relative eats" rather than "how they can lose weight"! It's never too late to listen to general advice about sensible eating and there are specific diets to help them improve poor appetite and gain energy.'

Diet is an important factor in any programme that is designed to build up strength and put back weight. A review of what your relative eats will be high on the list of changes that you can help them make. Dietary advice is readily available for patients, especially if your relative has undergone surgery of the gastro-intestinal tract. Talk to the practice nurse at the surgery who will have a selection of leaflets, and if you are unsure about how to make changes ask the doctor if your relative can be referred to a dietitian who will give specific advice tailored to their needs.

Some people inherit a tendency to be a certain shape and others gain or lose weight more readily than the next person. In basic terms, anyone who eats more, or fewer, calories than they burn up will usually go up or down in weight. The simple rules to controlling weight are: eat foods that are energy-rich to put on weight or foods that are calorie-reduced to lose weight. When helping your relative to cut back or increase calories it is important to keep an eye on the nutritional content of the diet and not reduce their intake of valuable vitamins and minerals. When appetites are 'picky' select foods that give a good value per calorie. For example, chocolate is one of the first things that overweight people avoid but it is a useful source of iron, fat and calories, in an easily digestible form, if your relative can eat very little.

Diana, a dietitian

'The good news is that a lot of benefit can be gained by making minor changes. It is important that your relative continues to enjoy food so don't make dramatic changes overnight – introduce new foods and cooking methods gradually and buy a variety of foods so that a healthy balance is maintained.'

Eating problems

People who are ill with cancer usually lose weight and they may have problems regaining their appetites. If this is affecting your relative, check the list below to identify the reasons why they might be struggling to regain an interest in food.

- Too tired to eat.
- Too weak to manage to feed themselves.
- Generally depressed and anxious.
- Difficulty swallowing food because their mouth is dry and sore or their throat is constricted.
- Dentures no longer fit properly.
- Indigestion after eating.
- Nausea and sickness because of chemo- or radiotherapy.
- Reduced stomach capacity.
- Constipation.
- Anxious about affecting their colostomy.
- Food tastes unpleasant.

Finding a solution

The dietary advice for many of the problems listed above is similar; however, if your relative has very marked or specific problems it may be best to seek professional help from a dietitian. For general self-help and pick-me-up tips, you could:

- ask them what foods would trigger their taste-buds, as small amounts of 'snack' type food may be better than a 'proper' meal;
- provide smaller meals on a small plate to avoid the overwhelming sight of a normal-sized helping;
- let your relative eat on request, when he or she feels peckish;
- pack meals with interest and nutritional value, attractively presented;
- keep food light – eating stodgy, hard-to-chew food saps energy quickly;
- avoid rich, spicy food if it causes nausea and irritates the digestive tract; conversely if your relative's taste is reduced, 'pep up' taste-buds with strongly flavoured foods;
- liquidise foods into easy-to-swallow drinks using milk or fruit juice as fluid;
- ensure food is moist as it's easier to eat than dry food and provide a bowl of crushed ice to keep the mouth wet – fruit flavoured tastes better;
- keep the freezer well stocked with a choice of refreshing ice-creams;
- try all-in-one meal drinks and use these as a drink after or instead of a meal (some makes are available on prescription);
- offer a straw if the mouth is sore or it's easier to drink lying down – a shorter straw needs less suction for very weak patients;
- ask the dietitian about granules that thicken liquids if too runny foods are a problem (cornflour and arrowroot work well at home);
- offer a glass of sherry as an *apéritif*;
- resist hassling your relative if they lose interest – a relaxed, 'no-problem' atmosphere is more likely to succeed;
- offer a little help (if it appears welcome) – cut up food into manageable-sized portions or feed your relative if they tire very easily;

■ sit with them for a bit and share a quiet meal – it's a good time to catch up on family news. Let them eat whilst you talk;

■ increase the fibre-rich/high residue foods if constipation is a problem and speak to your doctor, a pharmacist or nurse about laxatives. The high fibre products available today are far more gentle on the bowel than some 'opening' medicines that older people may ask for;

■ increase foods that bind the stools (reduced fibre/low residue foods) if diarrhoea is causing discomfort – and seek advice.

Build-up diet

This way of eating is devised to help cancer patients maintain or build up their weight. It means introducing foods high in energy and protein into the diet, with the emphasis on richness and increased calories. Many people with cancer experience eating problems at some point during the illness; however, everyone needs a certain level of energy to run their body, even if they are very inactive. Once treatment regimes are completed, your relative can be encouraged to overcome any difficulties and resume normal eating habits. A diet that is advised for someone who is losing weight, or to help increase weight, is designed especially for that job; it is not recommended long term for people who are eating well.

To help your relative build up their strength, choose a selection of foods regularly from the following lists when preparing meals, according to dietary need.

■ **High energy foods:** bread, pasta, cereals, cake, sweet biscuits, and glucose sweets.

■ **High protein foods:** meat, poultry, fish, beans, lentils, eggs, milk and cheese; however, to reduce the risk of infection, cook eggs well and avoid dairy products made from unpasteurised milk.

■ **Rich fatty foods:** oils, butter, margarine, fatty meats and oily fish, full-fat dairy products (for example, fresh cream), nuts and mayonnaise. Look for labels that state whole milk and full-fat rather than products that claim to contain low-fat or 'light' ingredients.

- **Vitamins and minerals:** whilst vitamins and minerals are contained in most foods, some of the best sources are raw or lightly cooked fruit and vegetables with skins intact.

If your relative is frail and has lost weight, you may need to use subtle ways to introduce extra goodness, without adding too much bulk.

- Add extra milk or cream to soups, puddings, custard, mashed potato, breakfast cereals and drinks in the form of fortified milk foods (available from pharmacies), evaporated or condensed milk or dried milk powder and use milk when the recipe states water.
- Add extra lentils, split peas, beans or egg noodles to meat stews and casseroles.
- Put a spoonful of real cream, rich ice-cream or condensed milk on to puddings.
- Use extra honey or syrup on breakfast cereals or porridge (made with milk or single cream).
- Keep a selection of nibbles, such as peanuts, crisps and dried fruits in handy dishes about the house.
- Spread butter, margarine and mayonnaise more thickly and add to mashed potato and vegetables.

Alternative diets

Unless it has been recommended by your relative's doctor, don't be tempted to make drastic changes in diet, as this is not the time to start experimenting with extreme, new diets; foods that taste good, that are familiar and comfortable to eat work best during times of stress. Alternative diets for treating cancer have been well publicised in the media over recent years. Examples include eating large amounts of vitamins or carrot juice. Unfortunately, there is little medical evidence that introducing intensive, strict regimes will prevent cancer or greatly improve the chances of recovery, and excessive consumption of certain vitamins (A and D) can be harmful. The standard advice for most cancer patients suggests that following a sound, nutritional diet will help boost the immune system and make dietary sense.

For more *i*nformation

i CancerBACUP booklet *Diet and the cancer patient* (address on page 261).

Alcohol

There is clear evidence that alcohol consumption is a trigger factor in the development of some cancers, particularly those that start in the digestive tract (see Chapter 1). The main message from doctors and scientists suggests that alcohol in small amounts may be beneficial and will do no obvious harm, for the majority of people. In the face of all the evidence from many studies throughout the world the most sensible advice is that alcohol should only be drunk in moderation. It is still strongly linked to many other causes of illness and death – liver disease, strokes, and accidental death. In general the recommended weekly amount for men is a maximum of 20 standard drinks. Women, who are less able to metabolise alcohol because of smaller liver capacity, are advised to drink up to 12 standard measures. Everyone is advised to restrict their drinking by having at least 2 to 3 alcohol-free days each week to give their bodies a rest.

Drinking alcohol during or following treatment for cancer may not be possible, or recommended, and the advice for cancer patients may be more definite. Alcohol is frequently advised against for people taking a range of drugs. If your relative is unsure, ask their doctor first before adopting any general guidelines about alcohol consumption, as each case is individual. However, if with the doctor's permission alcohol is not banned, the indications are that drinking small, well-controlled amounts may be very pleasurable, although it is better to avoid undiluted spirits or drinking on an empty tummy. Aim to stay well below the recommended levels for people without a health problem, and try to avoid situations where a large, rich meal is accompanied by several drinks.

Smoking

The facts about smoking

Mark, a GP

'Tobacco is the substance most linked to the development of lung cancer. It is a myth that smoking may not be harmful. The proven evidence from a large number of scientific studies shows that all forms of smoking damage health: cigarettes, cigars and pipes. It's never too late to feel the benefits of giving up, and it's one of the most effective changes that anyone who suffers from cancer can make to improve their health.'

The facts about smoking-related cancers make sobering reading, yet despite extensive health education programmes, media attention and general knowledge about the risks, a large number of people continue to smoke. Smoking is the biggest avoidable cause of premature death and ill health; the earlier a person starts to smoke the greater the danger of developing cancer. Figures from the Health Development Agency indicate that 30 per cent of all cancer deaths in the UK are caused by smoking and cigarette smokers greatly increase their risk of high blood pressure and are twice as likely as non-smokers to have a heart attack.

Fact box

■ Approximately 111,000 deaths in the UK annually are caused by smoking:
  – 30,000 from lung cancer;
  – 11,000 from cancer of the gullet, larynx, bladder, kidney, pancreas and cervix;
  – 70,000 from other smoking-related diseases, for example heart attack.

- Lung cancer is the commonest cancer in men and the second commonest in women.
- People who smoke 20 cigarettes a day are 20 times more likely to get lung cancer.
- People who combine smoking with drinking alcohol are more likely to get cancer of the throat.
- If 1,000 male adults in England and Wales who smoke were compared with other causes of premature deaths, it is estimated that:
  - 1 will be murdered;
  - 6 will die in a road accident;
  - 250 will die prematurely from an illness caused by tobacco.

Source: Health Development Agency

The culprits

Tobacco smoke contains many poisonous chemicals that play a significant part in triggering serious ill health. As well as various cancers such as respiratory tract and bladder it triggers the build up of atherosclerosis (the process that hardens and furs up the artery walls) and the chemical action makes the blood thicker, increasing the chance of blood clots. The most serious damage is caused by three main substances:

- **Coal tar** lines the tissues of the lungs causing irritation and inflammation. One of the main dangers comes from benzpyrene, a strongly carcinogenic hydrocarbon substance present in coal tar, that forms when tobacco is burnt. In addition to the carcinogenic effect, the sticky tar deposits damage lung function and reduce the amount of oxygen getting across to the blood stream, which can lead to chronic bronchitis and emphysema, two conditions that eventually contribute to heart failure.
- **Carbon monoxide** takes the place of some of the oxygen in the blood stream so that vital organs, including the heart, are

117

deprived of essential oxygen, reducing its efficiency as a pump; it also aggravates arterial disease contributing to high blood pressure.

■ **Nicotine** is an addictive substance that acts as a powerful mental depressant but its chief danger is its ability to act swiftly on artery walls causing them to contract very strongly. These muscle spasms vastly reduce the flow of blood to the heart muscle and are a major cause of angina, the heart disease.

Most people do understand that smoking is bad for their health, especially when a family member has developed a tobacco-related cancer. If the person you are caring for has been in hospital they will have been told about the dangers and may have already given up. The problem often lies, not in the acceptance that smoking was the culprit, but in the ability to actually give up. Quitting smoking is not an easy thing to do as long-term smokers are usually addicted to nicotine and may suffer severe withdrawal symptoms. A difficult time can be during convalescence when stress levels are increased by boredom, fear of recurrent illness and anxiety about the future. If the desire to smoke is very strong, be ready to offer encouragement as you can help in lots of ways.

Tips to help stop smoking

■ Listen to your relative and try not to criticise any lapses – be sympathetic but firm.

■ Don't suggest that your relative start smoking again – however irritable they become.

■ Talk to other ex-smokers or telephone the freephone helpline run by an independent charity **Quitline** (0800 002200) that provides confidential and practical advice for people wanting to give up smoking.

■ Change routines so that old habits don't make it easy to light up. Identify danger times/places and alter behaviour if necessary; for example, sit in a different chair, drink tea instead of coffee and change routines after a meal – all times when a cigarette may have been smoked.

- Offer plenty to drink as ex-smokers need to flush the chemicals out of their system – fruit juice is good as the vitamin C helps rid the body of nicotine.
- Suggest different forms of entertainment to help cope with the boredom, particularly activities using their hands.
- Offer plenty of praise and support but don't overdo the sympathy – some sensitive people may rather not be reminded. Ask which approach works best.
- Suggest that your relative tells people; that way family and friends won't smoke in his or her presence and, hopefully, won't tease their efforts.
- Talk about the benefits of quitting. For example, after a few days the sense of taste and smell begin to return; after a few weeks the lungs are cleaner and breathing becomes easier; and after a year the risk of a heart attack is reduced by 50 per cent.
- Highlight the money that is being saved and think of ways to treat yourselves!

Although the main message remains the encouragement to stop smoking, there are times when this can seem like 'closing the stable door after the horse has bolted'. If your relative has advanced cancer and a limited expectation of life, and smoking is one of the few things that bring them pleasure, then it would be unkind to deny this one source of comfort. However, there is no reason not to use the illness to emphasise to other family members the importance of stopping smoking and to discourage them from ever starting.

Exercise

Exercise is good news for everyone, even for people who are recovering from a serious illness. However, the level of physical activity that a person undertakes (including planned exercise) must be tailored to suit their capabilities. Information in a book can only be written in a general way, so before taking any form of exercise, particularly in the immediate post-operative period, all patients must check with their doctor first and be sure they understand what is suitable for them. As the carer you can help your relative to plan their exercise sensibly, perhaps with the advice of a physiotherapist who is skilled in rehabilitation and in helping people get the best from an exercise programme. Consider joining in – shared activity is much more enjoyable than exercising in isolation.

Ben, a sports centre manager

'It is never too late to derive some benefit from exercise, the advantages are well proven. Exercise helps improve physical strength, mobility and mental wellbeing. It's very good for reducing stress as it boosts the hormones which produce feelings of happiness and the movement gently relaxes muscle tension. Muscles work more smoothly, with less effort, if they are made to work regularly. The Health Development Agency recommend exercise that boosts the three S's – strength, suppleness and stamina – all within moderation.'

In the past people spent long periods in bed after a serious illness to allow the body to heal. Fortunately, this is no longer the practice and patients are encouraged to be more active at an earlier stage. Not all exercise need be strenuous, no one will suggest that your relative takes up hard jogging or squash. Start gently with a mild physical activity combined with lots of pleasure.

Exercising safely

Whichever activity your relative chooses, it's important to be aware of a few safety rules, even with permission from the doctor.

- Start the regime gradually and build up exertion levels at a rate that feels comfortable; no one should behave as if they are training for the Olympics.
- Don't exercise for at least two hours after a meal as the digestive system places an automatic demand on the blood supply to digest the food.

- Wear clothes that are loose and comfortable and shoes or trainers that provide adequate support.
- Never rush straight into the most strenuous part of the activity, start and stop at a gentle pace to allow muscles to warm up and cool down before and after exercise.
- Drink plenty of fluids, but not alcohol as this increases dehydration.
- Stop immediately if there are any signs of breathlessness, chest pains or feeling unwell in any way; if exercise has caused problems, however minor, it would be wise to inform the doctor before continuing with the programme.
- Even mild increases in exercise may cause **leg cramps** for some people, particularly if this is after a long period of illness in which little activity or exercise has been possible. Your relative's doctor will advise about taking exercise if leg cramps are painful.

Philip, a physiotherapist

'When starting to exercise after an illness, look at activities that get the body moving gently. Choose sports that are pleasurable, not games that are stressful and competitive. Start off cautiously because too great an effort may reduce enthusiasm. Muscles need to stretch gently so "start and finish slowly" is the simple rule that can be applied to all activities listed below.'

The following activities are classed as leisure hobbies rather than exercises for fitness fanatics; some can be done alone, some need a partner. If you would like to join a club look in the local *Yellow Pages* or ask for details at the library.

- **Walking** is a good choice if you have been inactive as it boosts stamina and allows fitness to build up at a steady rate. Walking needs no special equipment, it's free, relaxing and pleasurable if shared with a companion. If your relative has become very debilitated by their treatment they must start very gently, perhaps with regular short walks gradually increasing the pace and distance over a few weeks.

■ **Swimming** is a good exercise for people of all ages as it combines stamina, strength and suppleness. It is often described as the ideal activity and it's a great stress reducer and especially good for people who are overweight or have joint or back problems as the water supports the body. Most people live within reasonable distance of a swimming pool and the charges are often reduced for certain groups of people.

■ **Cycling** is another good exercise to improve on the three S's. It is recommended for people who are overweight and helps reduce stress as well as being enjoyable. Cycling in the fresh air is the best choice but an indoor cycle machine provides an alternative way to get pedalling.

■ **Golf** is a great energiser. It helps build up stamina and strength, provides fresh air and an opportunity to make new friends. Start off gently with a few holes and stop to enjoy the company and scenery.

■ **Bowling** is excellent for suppleness and relaxation. Your relative may like to join a club to get the best advantage from indoor and grass bowls and try the ten pin variety for some challenging fun.

■ **Badminton** is a fun game which suits all ages as long as partners of similar ability are matched. At club level it can be quite a vigorous sport, so encourage your relative to build up skills at a pace that is comfortable and check out with the doctor before starting this type of exercise.

■ **Exercise and dance** classes are readily available in most areas. Ask at a leisure centre about classes to suit your relative's age and ability level. Both types of exercise are good for stamina, strength and suppleness and dancing is especially relaxing and enjoyable.

■ **Yoga** is an excellent form of exercise to control movements and breathing and encourage muscle relaxation. It's good for suppleness and strengthens body muscles.

For more *i*nformation

i For details of local adult sport and leisure activity classes, contact the Community Education department at the local education authority or private leisure centres.

i Sport England provides general information about all sports (address on page 272).

i EXTEND provides recreational movement to music for older and less able people. EXTEND is active in many parts of the UK and trained teachers provide one-to-one sessions for those who require specialised exercise. Contact the address on page 265 for details of any local classes or teachers.

Sleeping well

Depression, tension and stress are common contributors to sleep problems, causing early waking or difficulty dropping off when thoughts race around the brain. If stress is making you or your relative sleep badly, don't rush for medication; instead, try practising the relaxation techniques described in Chapter 8. Be aware that older people naturally take longer to fall asleep, are more likely to wake during the night and tend to wake earlier in the morning. However, if sleep disturbance continues or if early waking is a problem do encourage your relative to discuss this with their doctor as these symptoms are a sign of depression which can be treated.

Tips to help settle at night

■ Go to bed at a regular time, with a regular routine.
■ Make everything as cosy as possible – a warm room and a comfortable bed.
■ Don't eat a rich, heavy meal late in the day.
■ Avoid stimulating drinks that contain alcohol or caffeine later in the day and choose a milky drink at bedtime.
■ Cut back on evening fluids if a full bladder is the cause of waking.

■ Read or listen to the radio until you naturally feel sleepy. If you wake in the night do the same or get up and watch some television and repeat the milky drink with a biscuit if you are feeling hungry – don't lie tossing and turning.

■ Take regular exercise, but don't be too active late in the day as strenuous exercise releases hormones that are stimulating.

■ Rest and cat-nap during the day but resist having too long a sleep as this simply reduces the amount needed at night.

Dealing with extreme tiredness

Fatigue is more than being 'tired', it is feeling completely exhausted most of the time. Extreme tiredness is a problem that almost all cancer patients experience at some time, particularly during treatment. Symptoms of fatigue may create difficulty in coping with the most basic, everyday activities such as climbing stairs, brushing teeth and eating food. Shortness of breath is common and many patients find it too arduous to carry on a conversation, concentrate to read or even watch the television.

Jill, cancer centre nurse

'Fatigue is made worse by a combination of factors related to illness and treatments – nausea and sickness, pain, poor appetite, lack of sleep, anxiety, depression, possible infection and anaemia may all contribute. Trying to battle against extreme weariness increases debility, so persuade your relative that for a while it may be easier to give in and let others take over the major tasks of shopping, laundry and household chores. Help your relative to plan their day so that they can achieve the things that are most important to them, with lots of rest periods in-between.'

For more *i*nformation

ⓘ CancerBACUP booklet *Coping with fatigue* (address on page 261).

Relationships

People who have known each other and/or lived together for a period of time often become very close after a diagnosis of cancer, offering each other tremendous support through the bad moments and sharing joy and relief when times are good. In the early days the illness may take over your lives and as a carer you probably feel in danger of being overwhelmed; the ill person gets all the attention and you are left coping with the practical and emotional difficulties. It may help to talk to a counsellor at this time and it also helps to keep a balance in your mind between what is necessary now for your relative against how you will return in the longer term to a more normal life.

Sexual feelings

When and how to resume sexual relationships after treatment is a sensitive issue for some people. If you and your partner have so far avoided the subject, choose an appropriate moment and broach the matter gently. It is important that you each have an opportunity to say how you are feeling. Emotions can cause severe anxiety, particularly following treatment for gynaecological cancer or disfiguring surgery. The sense of shock felt by either partner may be quite profound. Allow considerable time to overcome the trauma and build up trust to be sexually close again.

Molly, cancer nurse specialist

'People can express love for each other in many ways and being a carer as well as a partner is one clear example. But, however close you are to your partner, making the adjustment from a caring relationship back (or forward) into a sexual relationship may be a major step. A specialist nurse will not be embarrassed to discuss the matter and will be able to reassure you both; usually, there are few reasons to hinder a sexual relationship, if this is what you both want.'

The following suggestions offer helpful guidelines towards regaining feelings of self worth.

- Sexual pleasure can be achieved in many ways other than by direct sexual intercourse.
- Caressing someone gently is a non-threatening way to give and receive pleasure as the sense of touch rarely diminishes.
- The well partner should be prepared to accept less and give more in the early stages.
- Ask about, and tell, your partner what feels good.
- Spend time creating a relaxed atmosphere, show patience and offer reassurance.
- Buy a book from a reputable bookshop to learn more about sexual skills.
- Turn the light off and keep the bedcovers in place if this helps to dispel embarrassment.
- Be guided by your partner's mood and be careful about expressing negative feelings; a person who is struggling to cope with their own fragile emotions may not be able to handle yours as well.
- Be flexible about the time of day that you explore sexual pleasure – night time, after a tiring day, may not be best time to choose.
- Try different positions for love-making to ease any discomfort and put less strain on tired limbs.
- If problems persist after a reasonable time period, ask for advice from your specialist, GP or specialist nurse, they will either be able to advise you or help you to get more specialist advice if this would be useful.
- Telephone a specialist organisation for relevant literature; most cancer support organisations offer a range of leaflets (see 'Useful addresses' starting on page 258).

If your partner's cancer has not resulted in physical changes to sexual organs, the general advice after an illness is to treat sex like any other activity leading to recovery. Regular sexual relationships are beneficial in relieving tension and inducing feelings of wellbeing. Be wary of over-stressing operation scars and work on the principle that normal sex, with a known partner, puts a strain on the body equivalent to climbing two flights of stairs!

Impotence

> **John, a doctor**
>
> 'Male impotence may be a temporary problem following some types of treatment. If impotence is affecting your relative, do encourage him to seek help from a doctor as a range of treatments are available. A change of drugs or simple relaxation therapy may be all that is needed to improve the situation.'

Radiotherapy to the pelvic area should have no direct effect other than possible loss of sexual interest caused by tiredness; chemotherapy will probably have the same result. Information about infertility has been given in this book under the relevant treatment sections. Treatment for cancer of the prostate gland does often cause impotence so the doctor would discuss this with your relative before starting treatment, and also inform him of alternative options.

The doctor may ask if he has a morning erection as this information will help to define whether the cause is physical. Poor blood supply to the penis, leaking veins which cannot hold blood in the penis and the effects of certain drugs are all contributing factors that affect the quality of an erection, particularly in an older man.

For more *i*nformation

i CancerBACUP booklet *Sexuality and cancer* (address on page 261).

i SPOD: Association to Aid the Sexual and Personal Relationships of People with a Disability (address on page 272).

Signs of depression

Minor signs of depression, such as weeping and being withdrawn, are common after any serious illness, but persistent symptoms may indicate that your relative is developing clinical depression. Don't assume that the physical signs of depression – difficulty sleeping, early morning wakening, tiredness, poor appetite, lack of energy, feeling hopeless and worthless – are merely symptoms of post-cancer treatment. If you are concerned about possible depression do encourage your relative to talk to their GP. Treating depression after serious illness is common and helps rehabilitation. Talking and listening are excellent ways of starting self-help treatment.

Relieving boredom

Anne

'Tim was used to being busy and he did find it frustrating to have no energy. I bought a computer chess game which helped to reduce his boredom.'

There are many ways to lift the spirit and relieve boredom. Talk to your relative about the type of activities and company they would or would not enjoy. Get out of the house as soon as it is practicable to get a change of scene and overcome fears about leaving a safe place. Enlist the help of family and friends for all manner of support – from shopping and driving to companionship and listening. Try to gauge how your relative feels as you may need to act in a 'gatekeeping' role if offers of help are overwhelming.

The public library is the best source of information: most branches carry a wide range of details about local services, with some specialist facilities targeted at carers. As well as books of all sorts, look out for:

- lists of clubs and hobby groups;
- audio and video tapes;
- mobile and doorstep library services for home delivery of books and tapes to people who experience significant difficulty getting to a library because of illness, disability or caring responsibilities;

- 'Talking News' style services providing a range of interesting items via postal tapes, usually for visually impaired people but often extended to people with other disabilities;
- 'befrienders' schemes where volunteers come to the house to chat or play games with people who are temporarily or permanently housebound;
- branches of University of the Third Age (U3A) that offer a vast range of day-time study and recreational classes for people who are older and wish to keep their minds stimulated (address on page 273).

As your relative gains strength, suggest some active entertainment as well as the more passive type. A trip to an art gallery or an afternoon cinema programme may be just what's needed to trigger mental and social stimulation.

Anne and Tim

'We joined a French class at the local college as soon as Tim felt well enough to go out regularly and promised ourselves a holiday as a future goal.'

Transport

As recovery continues your relative may want to venture further from home, perhaps for a shopping trip or a hospital appointment, but travel may be a problem if driving is restricted or uncomfortable. Look out for transport schemes for older and disabled people, available in most areas, run by local authorities and voluntary organisations. The journey is free or subsidised, depending on personal circumstances and carers are welcome as escorts. Fares to hospital can be reimbursed for certain categories of people (see page 165).

The main schemes that help people with transport are listed below.

■ Dial-a-Ride and Community Transport Association schemes (address on page 262) provide door-to-door services for shopping or similar outings for people who cannot use public transport.

■ Hospital Car schemes are usually run by the ambulance service and arranged through GPs' surgeries. They are available only for people who have a medical condition and cannot get to the hospital independently; one companion is usually allowed.

■ The Orange/Blue Badge Scheme provides a national arrangement of parking concessions for people with severe walking difficulties who travel as drivers or passengers. Badge holders are exempted from certain parking restrictions, including free parking at on-street parking meters and for up to two hours on single and double yellow lines in England and Wales. Badges are issued for a three-year period through social services departments. Check local rules carefully as some London Boroughs do not offer free parking arrangements.

■ Motability (address on page 269) is a charity set up to help those disabled people who want to spend the mobility component of their Disability Living Allowance or War Pensioner's Mobility Supplement on a car, scooter or wheelchair. Vehicles may be purchased or leased and help may be available with the cost of special adaptations. A relative, friend or carer may apply and drive on behalf of a disabled person.

■ All train operators have a railcard that offers concessionary fares to disabled people, giving up to one-third off a range of rail tickets. An application form and booklet called *Rail Travel for Disabled Passengers* is available at most stations or from the Disabled Persons Railcard Office (address on page 264). All rail operators will give extra help to older or disabled travellers if they are notified in advance.

■ Shopmobility schemes provide free wheelchair/scooter loan services in many town centres for anyone with a mobility problem. Users can usually park free or be met at the bus station or taxi rank by prior arrangement. An escort service is often available for people who are visually impaired or wheelchair users.

■ Taxicard (or similar name) is a service providing subsidised taxi fares run by many local authorities for permanently disabled people who are unable to use public transport. One passenger may accompany the cardholder. Ask at your local town hall.

■ Tripscope offers a free nationwide travel and transport information and advice service for older and disabled people (address on page 273). Tripscope will help with planning a journey but it is not a travel agency so cannot make bookings.

■ The Community Transport Association has services to benefit providers of transport for people with mobility problems (address on page 262).

■ The Disability Benefits Centre (address on page 264) can provide information about exemption from road tax for vehicles used exclusively by or for disabled people receiving the higher rate of the mobility component of Disability Living Allowance (DLA) or War Pensioners' Mobility Supplement. You may claim on behalf of the person you look after by completing an application form from the Benefits Agency.

For more *i*nformation

❶ Age Concern Factsheet 26 *Travel information for older people.*

❶ Contact your local authority for more information about local schemes to help with transport.

Holidays

Jean

'We started off with a mini-break to build up our confidence. When that went OK, we felt safe to book a longer holiday.'

Once your relative is feeling better you may all benefit from a holiday. The GP will advise you about when the time is right and explain the main aspects of your relative's health care, especially if you are going abroad. At the planning stage it would be wise to find out about the following points in case you need to make special arrangements for:

■ taking drugs out of the country, principally controlled drugs for pain relief;

■ insurance cover because your relative has an existing illness;

■ dealing with the effects of heat and sunlight – or opt for a cooler climate.

Holiday planning services that specially deal with information for disabled people can be used, thus reducing much of the stress load. The organisations listed below are selected from the many companies that provide help.

For more *i*nformation

i Age Concern Factsheet 4 *Holidays for older people*.

i Air Transport Users Council publishes a booklet *Care in the Air* for disabled passengers (address on page 258).

i Helpbox is a computer database holding a comprehensive range of health-related information (address on page 266).

i Holiday Care Service provides information and advice on holidays, travel facilities and respite care available for people with disabilities, those on low incomes and people with special needs. A reservation helpline and holiday insurance information for disabled people are available (address on page 266).

i RADAR (Royal Association for Disability and Rehabilitation) provides information about many aspects of disability, including accessible destinations for holidays (address on page 271).

i Winged Fellowship Trust provides respite care and holidays for physically disabled people, with or without a partner, in purpose-built holiday centres and on overseas and touring holidays. Trained staff and volunteers provide care (address on page 274).

i Macmillan Cancer Relief (address on page 268) is sometimes able to give a grant towards paying for a holiday, under certain circumstances. It also runs a hotel for people with cancer.

i Disabled Living Centres Council will tell you of the Centre nearest you, where you can see and try out aids and equipment (address on page 264).

i Disabled Living Foundation provides information and advice about all aspects of daily living for people with disability (address on page 264).

i 'Family Doctor' booklets in a range of titles are available from most pharmacist/chemist shops.

i NHS Direct provides confidential health advice and information, 24 hours a day, seven days a week. The helplines are staffed by qualified nurses and health information advisors, who can offer immediate medical advice and reassurance. Tel: 0845 4647.

Conclusion

Sylvia and Derek

'Suffering a serious illness such as cancer results in many changes – don't give in and feel sorry for yourself. OK, so it might return but while you are feeling stronger make use of the time and do some of the things that you've promised yourself for years.'

This chapter has encouraged you to focus on some of the inevitable changes that are happening to you and your relative and has offered some hints about how to move forward. Adjusting to new situations is never easy, especially if the event that triggered the change was both distressful and beyond your control. We all deal with problems more effectively if we feel that an element of choice is involved and we are able to exercise some control over the situation. After a while, unpleasant memories do fade and you and your relative will be able to look ahead with greater confidence and perhaps benefit from changes in lifestyle. Whatever the long-term future holds, you will be able to access services when your relative needs more care. Chapter 8 provides an insight into causes of stress and offers some techniques to help you both cope whilst you adjust.

4 Being a carer

A 'carer' is defined as anyone who spends time and energy looking after another person who needs extra attention because of their age or physical or other disability. This could be a friend or neighbour but it is most likely to be a close relative. The word 'carer' in this context refers to an 'informal' or 'non-professional' person, rather than a trained worker. This chapter offers support and guidance to help you in your role of carer. Being a carer may present you with strong, emotional feelings and it may take a while to get used to the effect. Taking on a caring role is not something you set out to do, like a professional job with ample training – at least, not the sort of caring that you are doing now for someone you love. Most people start caring for someone with cancer in one of three ways: swiftly, following the dramatic diagnosis of an acute form of cancer; more gradually, because they have prepared themselves knowing their relative may suffer a relapse of an existing illness; and, lastly, the caring situation may develop over many years (even with cancer) as the health of a relative deteriorates. Whatever your experience has been, the way you became a carer will be special to you.

What does it mean to be a carer?

In general terms, caring varies from a full-time activity if someone is seriously ill to as little as keeping a regular eye on a relative's daily affairs. The aim of most carers is to help the less able person remain in their own home, leading as stress- free and independent a life for as long as is possible. Wherever your position on the spectrum of care, it's likely that you are undertaking many of the following tasks:

- providing a safe and comfortable home;
- doing practical jobs such as shopping, cooking, cleaning, laundry and gardening;
- giving personal care and doing basic nursing procedures;
- offering love, emotional support and company;
- providing help and advice on running personal affairs;
- reducing isolation and bringing a bit of the 'outside world' into the daily life of someone who may be terminally ill.

Fact box

Information published by Carers UK, for National Carers Week June 2001

- Nearly six million people in the UK look after a relative or friend who cannot manage without help because of sickness, age or disability.
- More women (14 per cent) than men (11 per cent) are carers.
- The peak age for becoming a carer is between 45 to 64 years (20 per cent of adults).
- Estimates suggest there may be 51,000 carers aged 16 years or under – most of them care for a parent.
- The financial support for carers is paltry – Invalid Care Allowance (available to certain carers) is one of the lowest welfare benefits of its kind.

- Carers provide support worth £34 billion a year, yet many are excluded from benefits.
- 53 per cent of carers who live in the same household as the people they care for reported that they were the only carer.
- CarersLine (see page 262) receives 20,000 enquiries per year..

Source: General Household Survey 1998

Recognising yourself as a carer

Jean

'When Robert was diagnosed with bowel cancer I felt numb with fear. I was so shocked I couldn't think about what to do next. When he came out of hospital, I never called myself a carer.'

You may not think of yourself as a carer because you undertake your tasks out of love and friendship and you may have fallen into the caring role because no-one else is available. Many carers do not recognise themselves as such and therefore do not seek information or know where to look for further help. Now that your relative has cancer it is vital that you are aware of the support and help that is available and also that you also have rights as a carer that go alongside the responsibilities. This chapter offers information, advice and support to anyone who cares in some way for a spouse, relative or friend. It cannot give you all the answers or solve all your problems but it may help you to understand better some of the issues faced by non-professional carers.

There are an estimated 5.7 million carers in the UK (one in eight people), nearly two million of whom provide substantial amounts of care. At times being a carer creates tremendous anxiety and distress;

you may be undertaking tasks that feel difficult and unfamiliar, you are largely unpaid and untrained, and are often on duty for 24 hours each day, seven days a week. You will need to pace yourself, use a range of skills and experience, take on an enduring commitment, build up strong physical and mental systems, control your emotions and maintain a good sense of humour. Quite a lot to expect from one person! This responsibility will tax your patience and you won't always get it right – life is never completely straightforward and you may feel that it has already dealt you a nasty blow – but there are many sources of support you can draw upon to help you cope with very difficult situations and find ways of managing the stress.

Your feelings as a carer

Tess, a carers' support worker

'Carers often feel tired and upset – these are normal reactions to the situation but if you begin to feel over-stressed, angry and weepy these powerful emotions may be a signal that you need a short break. I realise it's easy to say "be calm", but lots of emotional energy can be spent worrying when it won't actually help.'

You will have your ups and downs and there will be days when you feel you cannot cope. Even if you chose your caring situation without hesitation this will not stop you from having negative feelings, and whilst most people decide to care willingly this will not be true of every carer. Professional people who work with carers understand that carers feel a range of very conflicting emotions and that sometimes these spill over and are directed towards their relative and towards the people who offer them support. Anger, frustration, fear, resentment and guilt will often exist alongside other emotions such as sadness, love, anxiety and concern. Powerful emotions can drain and exhaust you so try not to add 'worry' to the list. Worry and guilt are two emotions that cause much wasted energy. Look instead at problems from a different angle – if you feel in control, you will cope well; if the problem is not within your control, spending time being worried or guilty won't improve the situation and may even prevent you finding a solution. Carers frequently bottle up strong emotions to protect others but you need an outlet yourself. Letting go of unhappy feelings is better than storing them up.

Sizing up the problem

It is still assumed in society today that a blood-tie or marriage relationship automatically makes a person (usually the woman in the partnership) the main carer and that in this role she must undertake a number of demanding, unpaid tasks. You may believe this yourself. It may be assumed by others that you have the ability to cope and that your capacity to care can stretch to meet all the demands that are placed upon you. You may feel that other people expect so much from you – family members, doctors, social workers and nurses – and that you cannot let them down.

To help you come to terms with your role as a carer, it's important that you think about all of these expectations – including what you expect of yourself. If you feel confused or overwhelmed by the enormity of the task, talking to someone, perhaps another carer or a counsellor from a cancer centre, might help. Look at the list below and tick off those feelings that have crossed your mind in recent weeks.

- I lack confidence and feel inadequate.
- I have no qualifications to do the job.
- I am worried about shortage of money.
- I lack recognition/status.
- I am not sure where to turn for allies or support.
- I am bewildered by the maze of services.
- I am unclear about what I can ask for.
- I feel my needs are always disregarded in favour of 'the patient'.
- I have no time or space to be myself.

These thoughts are very common, even if they have been only fleeting. Don't block them out. Accept that occasionally carers do feel unable to carry on and sometimes they are forced to take dramatic steps to make their voice heard. Support workers should do everything in their power to ease your position and avert a crisis. Unfortunately, not all carers have access to an adequate, informal support system. If this applies to you do speak to your GP or the duty social worker at your closest social services office and ask about additional help before crisis point is reached.

Setting boundaries

Angela, a carers' support worker

'Many people become carers without being aware that carers have rights to services and that they do have choices about their situation.'

How did you become a carer? Did it creep up on you slowly as your relative's health got worse or were you thrust into the role suddenly because of crisis? Whatever the original reason, at some point it is vital that you sit back and take stock of the current situation. Ask yourself a few searching questions and think logically and seriously about the answers. Telephone a helpline and talk to a counsellor (see 'Useful addresses' on pages 258–274); an unbiased listener may help you sort out your feelings.

Ask yourself:

- Why am I doing this job?
- Will I feel that I have rejected someone I love if I stop?
- Is the caring situation going to be long or short term?
- Am I being pressured by other people?
- Do I want to continue or pass the responsibility over to others?
- What are my options for change?

As a carer you must make a conscious decision about whether to continue with caring or not. Making a definite choice will increase your mental strength to cope with the task, however difficult. There may be times when carers feel in despair, but when they perceive that they have no choice, that they were pressured into the situation by others or that they did not fully consider the seriousness of the situation, they are more likely to become angry, resentful and suffer ill health. There is nothing wrong with saying 'no' if you already feel over-burdened. If you cannot continue to care for your relative at home, you can still continue to be involved with their day-to-day care.

How 'good' is your caring situation?

Rita

'As my mother's health got worse I took over more of the responsibility for her day-to-day care. I lived around the corner so it was easy to stop by on my way to and from work. We took each stage at a time and my mother and I talked honestly about how things were going.'

Researchers studying informal caring, given by close relatives, have identified a model of a good caring situation that is recognised by professional people as an important factor in maintaining a positive experience for the key people involved. Whilst acknowledging that no caring situation can hope to fulfil the ideal all of the time – especially if your relative is terminally ill – it is important that everyone accepts the value of such a model and works towards achieving some of the suggestions.

The model list

- The carer makes a conscious choice whether to care or not.
- The carer is able to recognise their own limits and needs.

- The carer lives close by, but not necessarily in the same house.
- A network of care is set up, so that responsibility is shared.
- The carer has time to themselves and doesn't have to give up most of their own life.
- The carer has access to information and help to learn skills.
- A good past relationship existed between the carer and the person being cared for.
- The dependent person wishes to stay as independent as possible.
- The dependent person retains their own friends.
- The carer fosters independence in the person they are caring for.
- Everybody keeps a sense of humour.
- Professional help is there when it is needed.
- The carer feels supported and valued.

What formal support is available for carers?

Increasingly, the rights and needs of carers are being taken into account, although it has taken many years of lobbying by pressure groups and individuals and changes in legislation to reach the stage we are at now. A number of Acts of Parliament have been passed, and local charters produced, to secure and highlight the rights of carers and disabled people. The most relevant pieces of legislation are summarised here. If you need a more detailed explanation of your rights and the services to which you are entitled, you should contact your local social services department (social work department in Scotland) which will be listed in the telephone directory.

State provision

NHS and Community Care Act 1990

The NHS and Community Care Act is designed to help meet the care needs of older people, those with learning and physical disabilities and mental health problems, preferably in their own home or the area where they live. Social services take the lead role and work together with the NHS and voluntary organisations to offer a broad range of services for people in need and their carers. The services cannot promise to meet all needs, because community care is subject to certain eligibility criteria (see pages 179 and 181) but a trained person, called a care manager, will assess the needs of the person you care for and then, if that person is eligible, arrange appropriate services in what is known as a 'care package'. The services (care package) arranged through social services are means tested.

Carers (Recognition and Services) Act 1995

This Act defines a carer as 'someone who provides (or intends to provide) a substantial amount of care on a regular basis', including children and young people under the age of 18 years. It contains two main elements that deal with the rights of carers: to ask for a separate assessment of their own care needs when the person they care for is being assessed or reassessed; and the duty of local authorities to take into consideration the findings of this assessment when deciding which services to offer the person being cared for (see Chapter 4).

The Act requires social services departments, if requested to do so by a carer, to assess the ability of a carer to provide and/or to continue to provide care, and take this care into account when deciding what services to provide to the person being cared for. To qualify for an assessment a carer must be providing (or intending to provide) regular and substantial care, and the person they care for must be being assessed by social services at the same time. Because there is no official definition of 'regular' and 'substantial', each caring situation will be assessed individually. The assessment should recognise the carer's knowledge of the person, and the responsibility for the caring situation should be agreed as a shared undertaking between the carer and the social services department.

A new act of parliament, the Carers and Disabled Childrens Act 2000, will provide carers with additional legal protection, but may also change local procedures relating to carers.

Carers UK

'The Carers' (Recognition and Services) Act 1995 has been one of the most significant developments in the history of the carers' movement. Not only did it recognise the rights of carers for the first time, but the campaign which led to the Carers Act showed the level of agreement there was about the rights and needs of carers.'

Charters

Most social services departments have drawn up charters which aim to tell people what they can expect from the agencies that provide 'community care' services for adults. For example:

Charters for carers usually acknowledge the valuable role carers perform in caring for someone at home. They state that practical help for carers is a key priority for social services departments and sets out how they aim to help carers. These Charters offer:

- Recognition for carers.
- Practical help.
- Information and advice.
- Advice on welfare benefits.
- A short break from caring.

Community care charters complement the Community Care Plan and are about the services that help people to remain in their own homes. They cover such areas as understanding people's needs; planning care; the services people can expect to receive and what to do if things go wrong.

Charters for long-term care (called *Better Care – Higher Standards*) cover such areas as home care services and personal help or care in nursing homes. They tell people what the local authority and health services can provide and how to get these services more easily.

Contact your social services office to find out about local charters.

143

Carers' support centres and workers

Teresa, carers' support worker

'Before you meet a professional person, jot down a few notes as it's important to ask the questions that are right for you. Try not to make assumptions about what you think may be available – people are often surprised at the amount of services that exist.'

There are many schemes set up around the country specifically to provide help and support for carers; they are run mainly by health and social services teams and voluntary organisations. The workers understand the problems and feelings of isolation experienced by carers and are specially trained to help carers receive relevant and up-to-date information, gain access to services and welfare benefits and guide them in their caring role. Support workers welcome contact with you as a carer and will listen to your hopes, concerns and fears. Many produce newsletters, run local support groups for carers and have drop-in and respite care facilities.

Angela, carers' support worker

'We understand that carers get to the end of their tether and may be quite close to physical and mental collapse at times; occasionally it is their relative who takes the brunt of their anxieties and anger. Tension is usually relieved through shouting but carers can lose their temper more violently. If you feel it's time to look at ways of relieving the strain then do seek help before you reach crisis point. If you feel really desperate then give the Samaritans a call.'

Your own needs as a carer

Margaret

'Although my husband's needs come first I do think about myself as well. If I couldn't function he would suffer so I try to rest when he is asleep and I sit with him and we eat together.'

Don't ignore your health and well-being. This may sound like a tall order but you do need to maintain your own strength.

- Eat regularly and properly. If you are preparing meals for someone else try not to skimp on your own food.
- Take regular breaks from caring, even if you only find time to walk in the garden or read a book. Plan longer breaks at regular intervals.
- Arrange time away from the house to meet other people because isolation can be a major problem for many carers. There are sitting services available that will send a volunteer to stay with your relative – try a local Age Concern.
- Learn to move your relative safely, because strained and injured backs are a great problem for carers who are suddenly thrust into a caring role. Ask your community nurse or social worker about how to do this.
- Take catnaps during the day if sleep at night is disturbed – without feeling guilty.
- Ask about help with housework or gardening if you are over-tired. Some local authorities and voluntary organisations run volunteer gardening schemes.

Talking about feelings

One of the difficulties faced by carers is how to talk to their relative about the cancer. Likewise, the problem of how to communicate with relatives may also be bothering the person with the cancer. In truth, cancer remains a topic that many people find hard to broach and are awkward at discussing. There seems to be a 'code' that governs where and when the subject is introduced – for example, not in front of the person with the cancer and not with younger children. Carers and cancer patients sometimes find it easier to introduce the subject with professional people than with their own family; however, even doctors and nurses are not always comfortable answering questions and giving information.

Many carers express a desire to simply 'talk to someone' but often they don't know where to start or even whether they ought to be discussing their relative's illness. But talking can be of great benefit, so if you dread the thought of talking about cancer try to overcome your reluctance and help each other to say what you each feel.

What can be gained by talking?

- Support for each other.
- Comfort and a sense of togetherness.
- Reduction of fear and isolation.
- Agreement on ground rules about behaviour and openness.
- A sense of perspective.
- Clarity and answers to questions.
- Regaining and/or retaining a sense of control.
- Sharing of information.
- Correction of myths.
- Finding solutions to problems.

The list could be longer – perhaps you and your relative can add some benefits that you have gained by talking about their cancer. If you need a listening ear from outside your immediate circle there are many other people and organisations to whom you can turn for support (see pages 89–90).

How to share feelings

Eva
'My husband and I are very close and we have never found it difficult to talk about issues – until he had cancer. Once we got over our reticence we both agreed that it was fear of the unknown that held us back.'

There are no rules or easy answers that help deal with the topic to make everyone feel less uncomfortable.

- Behave in a sensitive and responsible manner, agreeing that matters spoken about privately remain confidential and details will only be passed on with express permission. For example, you could say 'May I share this information with ...?'
- Let your relative set the pace if this feels easier.
- Acknowledge open emotions and be supportive, but don't attempt to stop the flow however upset the person seems to be.
- If you are having a bad day, try to express what the emotion feels like and why, for example 'I feel low today because ...' is much easier to understand than a withdrawn manner.
- Expression of strong emotions is neither right nor wrong – being offered the opportunity is important.
- Give each other a chance to respond and time for non-verbal actions. A good hug or sitting in shared silence may be enough.
- Don't be frightened of speaking about the past or the future.

For more *i*nformation

🛈 CancerBACUP *Who can ever understand? Talking about your cancer* (see page 261 for address)

Talking to children

Talking to children about the illness of a close relative will be a painful task that at least one family member must be prepared to take on. Children are often very perceptive and quickly pick up on family problems. However distressing it may be, it's better for the child to be told at an early stage and then kept informed. Ask a health professional for help if this would make the job easier as they can advise you about how to introduce the subject and about appropriate language. Talk to each child at a level that is right for their own emotional development, which may differ from other children in that age group. The person who speaks to the child should know them well because it's important to be aware of their reaction. It's also important to answer the child's questions truthfully and simply and to try and avoid euphemisms which children may misunderstand. Even very young children will be aware of serious illness in a parent or close family member and this needs simple explanation. Children need to know how the person's illness will affect their own life and routine, and where possible their routine should be disrupted as little as possible. It may be necessary to repeat the information several times and be prepared to return to the subject as often as the child wishes, however upsetting this may feel for the adult.

The child has the right to be treated with respect and to be covered by the same code of confidentiality afforded to adults. Wider family members should be aware that the child knows about the illness as the child may approach others for confirmation. It is not fair to give a child false hope or inaccurate information to save an adult distress so the information that is given should be honest and consistent. Take great care that the child knows that they are not to blame in any way for the illness – that cancer is a disease that affects many people and no one is at fault.

Children may also need special support and understanding in bereavement. Often this is difficult for those left behind to do as they can be so wrapped up in their own feelings. Special counselling is available to help children in bereavement; your specialist palliative care nurse, GP or health visitor should be able to tell you what is available in your area.

For more *i*nformation

ℹ️ CancerBACUP leaflet *What do I tell the children?* (see page 261 for address).

ℹ️ Cancerlink leaflet *Talking to children when an adult has cancer*, available from Macmillan Cancer Relief at the address on page 268.

ℹ️ Cruse Bereavement Care (address on page 263) offers bereavement counselling for children.

Respite care and practical support

Much help is provided to carers by the hospices and specialist palliative care services (see Chapters 6 and 7). Most hospices offer respite to carers, either through admission, day-care or hospice at home, or Marie Curie nurses. They are able to offer psychological or emotional support to carers, and help guide them through the maze that the social services department can seem like. Also, there are many self-help groups and voluntary organisations who can offer considerable support to carers, as well as specialist support groups for certain cancers.

Practical support is also important and advice about where to get pieces of equipment sometimes gets overlooked because the professional person is focusing on the patient and may assume that the carer knows. Information and practical guidance about such procedures as moving your relative safely are best covered by the appropriate professional person at the time of need. Examples of useful caring aids is included in Chapter 6. If you are unsure about where to go for equipment or feel you do not have the skills to undertake a nursing task, do ask for help rather than continue to struggle.

Emergency help and first aid

Carers often express fears about what to do if there is an accident and their relative falls. The advice from the Ambulance Service is

149

dial 999 for help. Do not attempt to move the person as they will need to be assessed for injury.

If a situation occurs that needs prompt first aid, try to think and act calmly – you will be more effective and better able to reassure your relative. If your relative falls, collapses or becomes seriously ill, either call an ambulance yourself or ask someone to do this for you. Then treat your relative according to their state of consciousness, until help arrives.

If conscious:

■ Reassure your relative that help is on the way.
■ If your relative has difficulty breathing or complains of chest pains, gently raise them to a half-sitting position, with the head and shoulders supported.
■ If your relative feels faint, make sure that they are lying down, encourage them to take a few deep breaths but not to over-breathe because this can quickly cause dizziness for other reasons.
■ If your relative has fallen, do not move them unnecessarily as this may cause further injury.
■ If your relative has diabetes (as well as cancer) give them a sugary drink or a sugar lump or other sweet food.
■ Do *not* give anything to eat or drink if your relative does not have diabetes.

If unconscious:

■ If possible, lie your relative on the floor on their side; otherwise try to position the head with the jaw forwards in order to maintain a clear airway and to prevent saliva and the tongue falling backwards.
■ Remove dentures.
■ Loosen tight clothing.
■ Cover your relative with a blanket to keep warm.
■ Do not give any food or fluids of any kind.

If you become ill or need extra help

If you are ill yourself and need additional help at home during the day, you can contact the duty social services officer or your GP. For assistance outside office hours, contact the social services emergency duty team or a medical answering service. (Look up the numbers in the telephone directory and put them by the telephone now.)

Carer's emergency card

You might be concerned that you could have an accident or be taken ill while you are away from home, leaving the person you care for alone. You can obtain an emergency identity card that gives information about you as a carer so that your relative will not be left unattended. Cards are available from Carers UK (address on page 262).

Carers' advice line

A telephone helpline offering a wide range of information to carers operates nationally for the cost of a local call. Run by Carers UK, lines are open Monday to Friday from 10.00am to 12.00pm and 2.00 to 4.00pm (see page 262).

Emergency help systems

Many local authorities and some charities operate an emergency call system that is linked via the telephone to specially trained operators. (It may not be available to everyone.) A charge is usually made to help fund the system, which will vary from area to area.

For more *i*nformation

i Age Concern Factsheet 6 *Finding help at home.*

i Age Concern Factsheet 28 *Help with telephones.*

ⓘ Carers UK acts as the national voice of carers, raising awareness and providing support, advice and a range of information booklets. See page 262 for CarersLine and address.

ⓘ Counsel and Care (address on page 263) offers free counselling, information and advice for older people and carers, including specialist advice about using independent agencies and the administration of trust funds for single payments, for example for respite care.

ⓘ Books are regularly published offering information and support for carers. Check with support organisations for an up-to-date booklist or ask at your local bookshop.

Fact box

Information taken from *Facts about Carers* published by Carers UK.

- 1.7 million carers (27 per cent of whom are aged 65 years or over) do so for 20 hours or more every week – an increase from 1.5 million in 1990.
- 15 per cent of carers do so for over 50 hours per week.
- 71 per cent of those cared for are aged 65 years or over.
- 10 per cent of carers are aged 30 to 44; 13 per cent are aged over 65.
- 31 per cent of carers provide personal care; 27 per cent administer medicines; 73 per cent give other practical help.

Source: General Household Survey 1998

Conclusion

This chapter has offered material to help you focus on your role as the carer and given you an insight into the nature of caring. Reading the information may have been painful for you, especially if it raised uncomfortable questions that you found difficult to answer. If you are one of the many carers who are unfamiliar with the official system, hopefully it will encourage you to seek support and ask for an assessment of your caring situation. The statistics in the 'Fact boxes' show that you are not alone in the caring business. Take heart in the fact that the predicament of carers is now under open discussion and their efforts are being increasingly recognised and supported. This chapter has focused more on 'talking-style' support; subsequent chapters deal with everyday affairs and practical issues.

5 Dealing with practical and personal affairs

Helping to manage the financial and legal affairs of another person is one of the main roles of a carer. This may be because your relative has become too physically disabled or mentally confused to manage alone; because they feel unsure about dealing with people in 'authority' or because they no longer feel able to take decisions alone about complex issues. The timespan involved in taking over responsibility may be gradual or swift depending on the state of health and wishes of your relative.

This chapter outlines the services and agencies you could turn to for help and describes some of the welfare benefits and legal procedures that you and your relative may wish to investigate. It is unlikely that you will require all of the information at any one time but you can return to the relevant sections as necessary during your relative's illness.

Dealing with the affairs of another person is a serious business and you may feel daunted at first. However, there are people who will help you and there are many safeguards in place to protect you and your relative. Always cover yourself by seeking advice from a reputable source – a solicitor, an accountant, a bank or a voluntary organisation – before entering into legal contracts or making major decisions, especially concerning property or the management of your relative's money.

Eva

'After my husband was diagnosed with lung cancer I took over the financial affairs. The accountant did our tax self-assessment forms and I talked to the financial advisor about his health insurance policy.'

Finding out about help and advice

Getting the right information needs mental stamina, creative thinking and the investigative skills of Sherlock Holmes – or so it feels on occasions, particularly if you are tied to the house. With perseverance, however, you can be well informed. Look out for informative articles published by the local and national press and programmes broadcast on radio and television. The material is mostly well researched and aimed at the general public. For more detailed information, advice and advocacy there are many local and national organisations that offer carers a service; some are specialists in their field and others provide general information and act as signposts to the specialists. Most organisations offer facilities for disabled people and some information in minority languages. If time is precious ask a friend to investigate on your behalf. The main agencies to contact are listed in the Table below.

Roger

'Vera had always done the day-to-day household finances so when she wasn't up to it I had to think about budgeting the money. To save myself a journey to the post office I changed our pensions to go straight into our bank account and set up monthly payments for all the main bills.'

Jean

'When my husband was ill I got in a bit of a muddle paying the bills so my neighbour went with me to the Citizens Advice Bureau and they quickly helped me sort it out.'

Organisation	Services offered	How to contact
Advocacy services	Independent organisations in most areas that support and develop citizen advocacy work with people who need help controlling their affairs.	Local telephone directory or ask at Citizens Advice Bureau (CAB)
Age Concern	Can provide information, support, practical help, social activities and a range of publications for older people and carers.	Local telephone directory or address on page 275
Citizens Advice Bureaux (CAB)	Free, confidential advice and information on a wide range of legal, financial, social and consumer problems and help with form-filling and representation at hearings.	Local telephone directory
Counsel and Care	Provides free counselling, information and advice for older people and carers including specialist advice about using independent agencies. Publishes a range of factsheets and administers trust funds that make payments for equipment and respite care.	Address on page 263
Disability Information Services (called DIAL in some areas)	Advice on aids, equipment and services.	Local telephone directory
Disabled Living Centres Council	Advice on aids and equipment.	Address on page 264

continued

Organisation	Services offered	How to contact
Disability Living Foundation	Advice on aids and equipment.	Address on page 264
Jobseeker Plus/ Pension Service (formerly the Benefits Agency)	Provides information on welfare benefits and processes most local claims.	Local telephone directory
Benefits Enquiry Freephone	Provides general advice, information, claim forms and leaflets for disabled people and their carers by telephone or post but cannot deal with individual claims.	Tel: 0800 88 22 00 Minicom: 0800 24 33 55
Independent benefits advice agencies	Independent organisations in many urban areas and some rural areas offering free advice on problems relating to benefits, debt and work issues.	Local telephone directory
Help the Aged	Provides a range of services including Seniorline (a free information helpline).	Address on page 265
Housing advice	Many local councils provide a housing advice service to local residents in private or rented accommodation.	Local telephone directory
Hospice Information Service	Many hospices and specialist palliative care services often have either a welfare rights officer or social work team. Contact Hospice Information Service for details of your nearest service.	Address on page 266

continued

Organisation	Services offered	How to contact
Public library	Excellent source of local information, books, videos, directories, quality journals and many daily newspapers.	Personal visit, telephone, or limited home delivery
Neighbourhood schemes	Many local councils run community schemes offering a range of information and support to local people.	Local telephone directory under 'Council'
NHS Direct	Provides confidential health advice and information, 24 hours a day, seven days a week. Helplines are staffed by qualified nurses and health information advisors.	Tel: 0845 4647

State benefits and grants

The benefits system is complex and can only be covered broadly here because each person has individual needs and the information, amounts given and eligibility is subject to change. **The Department for Work and Pensions** (**DWP**, formerly the Department of Social Security) is the Government department responsible for social security. The administration of benefits used to be dealt with by the Benefits Agency, but this has now been replaced by Jobseeker Plus (benefits for people of working age) and the Pension Service (for pensioners). The range of benefits is listed in leaflets available from the DWP, most local authorities, Citizens Advice Bureaux and some post offices. Useful ones to look out for are:

■ DWP leaflet SD 4 *Caring for Someone*, which includes carers' benefits.
■ DWP leaflet SD1 *Sick or Disabled?*
■ DWP leaflet JSAL5 *Jobseeker's Allowance*.

For telephone advice about claims and information contact the local **Jobseeker Plus** or **Pension Service** office or the **Benefits Enquiry Freephone** (see page 158). If you need information about benefits in other languages contact your local DWP office.

People claiming a benefit must meet strict criteria; some benefits are means-tested or taxed or both. If you or your relative disagree with a decision made by the DWP, you have the right to appeal and ask for your case to be looked at again.

Benefits advisor

'Ask about benefits or you won't know what is currently available. It's really worth getting a knowledgeable person to check out your circumstances. Ask for help at the Citizens Advice Bureau.'

Why people are reluctant to claim

There are millions of pounds of unclaimed benefits, particularly those targeted at older people. Benefits advisors say that older people and carers are reluctant to claim means-tested benefits and many carers claim on behalf of a relative without realising that they might be eligible for benefits in their own right. The list below gives some reasons why eligible people do not make a claim:

- they think they are not entitled to money;
- they don't know what is available;
- they don't want to be bothered with the paperwork;
- they find the claim forms too complicated;
- they are too proud and believe that they may be taking money from someone else who is more deserving.

Benefits advisor

'Many older people and carers say that they feel too tired and busy to think about benefits. They continue to struggle and try to manage when they may be entitled to make a claim; it's OK to ask for help.'

159

Benefits for older and/or disabled people

Attendance Allowance

Attendance Allowance is for people aged 65 years or over who need help with personal care or someone to watch over them. It is tax-free and not means-tested but to qualify the person must normally have needed help with personal care for a period of six months. If Attendance Allowance is granted, it will be backdated to the date of claim, provided the six month qualifying period has been satisfied. However, people who are terminally ill qualify immediately. There are two rates according to how much care is needed. Get a claim pack from the DWP office or by calling the Benefits Enquiry Line (see the table on page 158). You could also contact one of the advice agencies (such as the Citizens Advice Bureau) which may be able to help your relative fill it in. (Leaflet DS 702.)

Disability Living Allowance (DLA)

Disability Living Allowance is for people who claim before 65 years of age and who have needed care or had mobility difficulties for more than three months. It has a care component for people who need help with personal care supervision or someone to watch over them, and a mobility component for people who need help with getting around. Disability Living Allowance is tax-free and not means-tested and not dependent on National Insurance contributions. The person receiving the allowance is free to spend the money however they choose; it does not have to be spent on care. The mobility component has two rates and the care component three; these are awarded according to the needs of the disabled person. People who are terminally ill qualify immediately for the highest rate of the care component. The Disability Living Allowance is a gateway to other types of help (for example the Orange/Blue Badge scheme, which gives holders special parking privileges). (Leaflet DS 704.)

Incapacity Benefit (IB)

Incapacity Benefit is for people under state pension age who are unable to work because of an illness or disability and have paid enough National Insurance contributions. The benefit is given at different rates, depending on how long someone has been unable to work. For the first 28 weeks, a claimant is assessed on their ability to carry out their own job, based on information given on medical certificates provided by the GP. After 28 weeks the sick or disabled person is assessed on how well they can carry out a range of work-related activities, called the Personal Capability Assessment. This assessment is carried out by completion of a questionnaire by the claimant and possibly also an examination by an appointed doctor. Some people may qualify for extra money if their husband or wife is over 60 years or they have dependent children. (Leaflet IB 1.)

Benefits for carers

Invalid Care Allowance (ICA)

To qualify for Invalid Care Allowance you must be providing care for at least 35 hours per week to a person who is receiving Attendance Allowance or Constant Attendance Allowance or the middle or highest rates of the care component of Disability Living Allowance. You must be aged 16 or over and under 65 years when you first claim (however, the upper age limit is to be abolished). You cannot get Invalid Care Allowance if you are in full-time education. You can have a job and still get Invalid Care Allowance but must not earn above a certain amount (after deduction of allowable expenses). The allowance is taxable. You may be able to get help with the cost of another carer if you work and you may be able to get extra money added to Income Support, income-based Jobseekers's Allowance, Housing Benefit and Council Tax benefit. Invalid Care Allowance can be backdated for three months. (Leaflet DS 700.)

Home Responsibilities Protection

Home Responsibilities Protection is not a benefit but a scheme which helps protect your basic Retirement Pension. If you are unable to pay National Insurance contributions or have not paid enough for any year of caring, you can apply for Home Responsibilities Protection, which helps towards qualifying for Retirement Pension. If you receive Invalid Care Allowance, you are entitled to National Insurance credits and will not usually need Home Responsibilities Protection. If you get Income Support because you are caring for someone, you will usually get Home Responsibilities Protection automatically. If you cannot claim Invalid Care Allowance for any reason but still care for over 35 hours per week for someone who receives Attendance Allowance, Constant Attendance Allowance or high or middle rate of the care component of Disability Living Allowance, you may be able to get Home Responsibilities Protection. (Form CF411.)

General benefits

Income Support (Minimum Income Guarantee)

Income Support is a means-tested benefit paid to someone aged 16 years or over whose income is below a certain level and who is not expected to sign on as unemployed. For people aged over 60 years the levels are higher and the benefit is called 'Minimum Income Guarantee'. The person must be incapable of work because of sickness or disability, or bringing up children alone, or aged 60 years and over, or registered blind or looking after a disabled person. Some people who are not in these groups may also qualify for help: Income Support can be paid to top-up other benefits or earnings from part-time work (including self-employment), provided they work fewer than 16 hours per week or have no form of income, or have not paid enough National Insurance contributions. Qualifications for Income Support may be affected by the level of their savings. (Leaflet IS 1.)

Jobseeker's Allowance

Jobseeker's Allowance has replaced Unemployment Benefit and Income Support for unemployed people looking for work. The allowance is paid to someone capable of working at least 40 hours per week who has paid sufficient National Insurance contributions or has income and savings below a certain level. The person must be resident in the UK, aged between 18 years and state pension age, and not in relevant education (for example, a full-time student). Although the person must be essentially unemployed and actively seeking work, some income may be earned from part-time work before Jobseeker's Allowance is affected. People claiming this allowance enter into a Jobseeker's Agreement. When drawing up this agreement, the adviser at the Job Centre will take into account any part-time voluntary work. (Leaflet JSAL5.)

The Social Fund

The Social Fund provides discretionary grants and loans to help people with expenses that are difficult to pay from their regular income. (Leaflet GL18 covers the benefits listed below.)

Budgeting Loans may be available to people receiving Income Support or income-based Jobseeker's Allowance (for at least 26 weeks) to help spread the cost of important expenses. Interest-free loans (which have to be paid back) may be available for specific items, such as furniture or clothing or to pay travel expenses.

Crisis Loans are for people with no savings or access to funds to help them cope with an emergency or disaster, such as fire or burglary, that puts the family at serious health or safety risk. Applicants do not have to be in receipt of other benefits. The interest-free loan has to be paid back.

Cold Weather Payments are paid automatically to some recipients of Income Support, including pensioners and disabled people, when the actual or forecast temperature goes down to freezing (zero degrees Celsius) or below for seven consecutive days.

163

Winter Fuel Payment is a one-off annual payment towards the heaviest winter fuel bill. It is normally paid automatically to most people aged 60 or over although some need to make an application.

Funeral Payments Help for funeral expenses is available to some people receiving means-tested benefits, who are responsible for the funeral of a partner, close relative or close friend. The payment may have to be repaid from any money or property left by the person who died. The DWP must agree that it is reasonable for the person to be responsible for the funeral before they will agree any payment, so people should check before making arrangements.

Bereavement Benefits People widowed below pension age may be entitled to bereavement benefits such as the Bereavement Payment or Bereavement Allowance. (Leaflet GL14.)

Housing Benefit and Council Tax Benefit

These benefits are worked out in a similar way to Income Support but are administered by the local Council (see below). Savings and income may affect how much you or your relative can get. Housing Benefit helps tenants pay rent and Council Tax Benefit helps tenants and home owners pay their Council Tax. People receiving Income Support and who claim Housing Benefit or Council Tax Benefit will generally automatically be awarded the maximum amounts. (Leaflet RR2.)

For more *i*nformation

ℹ️ Age Concern Factsheet 16 *Income related benefits: income and capital.*

ℹ️ Age Concern Factsheet 17 *Housing Benefit and Council Tax Benefit.*

ℹ️ Age Concern Factsheet 18 *A brief guide to money benefits.*

ℹ️ Age Concern Factsheet 25 *Income Support (Minimum Income Guarantee) and the Social Fund.*

ℹ️ Age Concern Factsheet 34 *Attendance Allowance and Disability Living Allowance.*

NHS benefits

A range of health-related benefits are available for people who receive other state benefits or are on a low income. These might help your relative with charges for prescriptions, eye tests and glasses, dentures and dental treatment, wigs and fabric supports and fares to hospital to receive NHS treatment. Some people (such as those on Income Support) are automatically exempted from some of these charges. Other people on a low income may get help if they apply on form HC1 (except for fares to hospital, which must be claimed from the hospital at each visit). Ask for details at your surgery, hospital clinic or a pharmacy.

For more *i*nformation

ⓘ Advisor's Guide to Help with Health Costs (NHS booklet: HC13).

Taxation

Inland Revenue

Home visits can be arranged for enquiries about personal income and other taxes if your relative is unable to get to a local office. A range of information is available in booklets, many of which appear in other languages, Braille and large print, and on audio cassettes.

Council Tax

Council Tax, collected by local authorities as a contribution towards local services, is assessed according to the value of each property and the number of adults in it. There are reductions, discounts and exemptions available that may help you as a carer and your relative. These relate to empty dwellings (you may have left your home to go and care for your relative or they may have moved in with you), to homes with substantial adaptations that are placed in a lower valuation band, and to people whose presence in a household is disregarded, so leading to a lower bill. Once your Council Tax liability is assessed you or your relative may be able to claim Council Tax Benefit (see above) to help pay. Get help from an advice agency (see the table starting on page 156) or your local authority.

For more *i*nformation

i Age Concern Factsheet 15 *Income tax and older people.*

i Age Concern Factsheet 21 *Council Tax and older people.*

Grants from private organisations

Many charitable trusts and foundations offer grants to help purchase one-off items of equipment, or pay for respite care. The qualifying criteria vary; for example, a trust fund may be open only to certain categories of people living in a defined area. Many cancer charities provide grants. For information about local and national grant-making organisations try asking at the hospice or cancer centre, the Citizens Advice Bureau, or the public library, or contact Counsel and Care (address on page 263) or the National Association of Councils for Voluntary Service (address on page 269). Occasionally parish councils administer minor trusts connected to a local benefactor.

Managing somebody's financial affairs

There are several ways that you can take over responsibility for your relative's financial affairs, depending on their physical and mental health status. Their needs may alter rapidly so be ready to increase your level of responsibility and be sure you have set up appropriate procedures before it becomes too late to make changes.

- **Agent** If your relative is mentally capable, but unable to get out, they can retain overall responsibility for their money but appoint you as their agent. You would be able to cash any pensions and benefits and you may be able to arrange a third party mandate to enable you to deal with bank and building society accounts on their behalf. Ask for details at a post office or bank, as many organisations have a standard application form.

- **Powers of attorney** If your relative has financial affairs, you may have to consider a power of attorney, which is a legal procedure to enable you to deal with their money. The **ordinary power of attorney** can be set up for cases where the person is able to give sound instructions; however, it will become invalid if the person becomes mentally incapable. To avoid this problem, most solicitors suggest an **enduring power of attorney** which can continue to be used even if your relative becomes too confused to manage their own affairs, provided it is registered with the Public Guardianship Office. It is important that you each take independent advice before setting this up, as it carries a heavy responsibility for the carer that could involve selling property and dealing with taxation. The procedure is very formal so, although not essential, it's usual to act through a solicitor. Further information can be obtained from the Public Guardianship Office at the address on page 270.

- **Court of Protection** If your relative is already 'mentally incapable', the action you can take will depend on their income. For state benefits only, you can become their **appointee**, a procedure that allows you to manage everything to do with their benefits. If the situation is more complex and you do not already have enduring power of attorney you can apply to the **Court of Protection**. They will appoint a receiver (usually a relative) to manage all the financial business. If you do not wish to undertake this duty, a bank or solicitor will act as receiver in your place. Contact the Customer Services Unit of the Public Guardianship Office (address on page 270).

Managing financial affairs in Scotland

The arrangements for managing someone else's affairs are different in Scotland. The Adults with Incapacity (Scotland) Act 2000 changed the system for protecting the rights and interests of adults who are incapable of managing their own affairs. It deals with the management of their property, financial affairs and personal welfare, including medical treatment. Many regulations and codes of practice have been introduced to deal with the matters raised in the new Act. The Public Guardian, an officer of the courts, supervises people exercising financial powers under the Act and keeps a register of those having powers of attorney.

It would be advisable for you and your relative to consult a solicitor, or approach your local Citizens Advice Bureau for advice.

For more *i*nformation

ⓘ Age Concern Factsheet 22S *Legal arrangements for managing financial affairs*, available from Age Concern Scotland (address on page 275).

ⓘ The Office of the Public Guardian provides an information pack that includes guidance notes and registration forms for powers of attorney, and application forms for authority to access and transfer funds (address on page 270).

ⓘ *Dementia, money and legal matters: a guide for carers*, published by the Accountant of Court, is available free to carers from Alzheimer Scotland – Action on Dementia (address on page 258).

Making a will

When someone is ill, they begin to think more about their personal affairs and may ask you to help them sort out the legal arrangements. Your relative may talk to you about making a will, or they may wish to add to or alter an existing will, if their situation has changed. If you feel uncomfortable or unsure about doing this task, ask someone else to help – perhaps a friend who is sensible and practical but less personally involved. If your relative is unable to go out, many solicitors offer a home service to help people write a will. Look in the *Yellow Pages* or ask at the Citizens Advice Bureau for details.

Some people draw up their own wills. This is quite in order as long as the correct procedures are followed. The will must be written clearly, and signed and dated in the presence of two (or just one in Scotland) independent witnesses or relatives who are not beneficiaries or married to a beneficiary. The will should name one or more people who are willing to act as executors – the people responsible for seeing that the instructions written in the will are properly carried out. Executors can be relatives, friends or professional people, who provide this service as part of their job (such as an accountant or a solicitor). A person who acts as an executor can also be named in the will as a beneficiary. Information packs and will forms are available from most stationers, and details of other booklets are given below. (If you live in Scotland make sure that the information covers the law in Scotland.) If your relative's affairs are not simple or straightforward, it would be wise to ask a solicitor to draw up the will; their fees for home and office appointments vary, so telephone and ask for a price guide before booking a home visit.

Why is a will important?

Some people wrongly assume that if their affairs are straightforward they do not need to make a will, because all of their belongings will go directly to their closest relative. But there are strict laws about how a person's estate (the name given to their possessions) is divided up and it can be complicated and costly to sort out the affairs of someone who has not made a will (called being intestate).

The following sensible comments from a solicitor should help if your relative is undecided and asks your opinion about the benefits of making a will:

- 'You don't have to have a lot of money to make a will. Making a will is about making sure that your possessions go to the person(s) you want to receive them.'
- 'You mustn't feel morbid about making a will; all you are doing is setting out your plan as to how your assets are to be split up when you die.'
- 'If you do not make a will the rules governing intestacy apply; which may mean that your assets will be given to relatives you do not know or even want to know.'
- 'Just saying to someone that a treasured ornament or a piece of jewellery is theirs when you die is not good enough. The only safe way of making sure that happens is to put it in a will.'

Registering a death

A death should be registered in the district where the death occurred, within five days unless the Registrar says this period can be extended. The person registering the death can make a formal declaration giving all the details required in any registration district in England and Wales. This will then be passed on to the registrar for the district where the death occurred who will issue the death certificate and any other documents. (In Scotland, it can be registered in the office for the area where the deceased person normally lived.) Some offices operate an appointment system, so telephone as soon as you receive the Medical Certificate of Cause of Death. Whether the death occurs in a hospice or at home you will be given the same type of Certificate. The address and telephone number of the local office are in the telephone directory; leaflets are available from the office.

In certain circumstances the death will be referred to the Coroner; if this is the case you will be advised what to do. A Coroner is usually involved when the death is sudden, unnatural, unexplained or attended by suspicious circumstances. A common reason is because the GP has not seen the deceased within the last 14 days.

It is usual for the death to be registered by a relative but it can be another person. Allow a reasonable amount of time to complete the formalities and it helps to have certain pieces of information to hand. The Registrar will want to know the following information about the deceased person:

- the date and place of death;
- their full name (and maiden name if appropriate);
- their date and place of birth;
- their occupation and that of the husband for a married woman or widow;
- their usual address;
- whether they were in receipt of a pension from public funds;
- the date of birth of their spouse if appropriate;
- their NHS number or actual medical card if available.

Certificates

There are three types of certificates issued by the Registrar depending on who must be told of the death. By law a Registrar cannot issue the necessary Certificates unless he or she is certain beyond all reasonable doubt that the death is above suspicion, particularly if the body is to be cremated.

- **A Certificate for Burial or Cremation (Green Form)** is supplied for the funeral director. He or she cannot proceed without this document. This certificate is free of charge.
- **A Certificate of Registration of Death** is supplied for social security purposes. Relatives are asked to read the details on the reverse of the form and return it to the local DWP office if particular circumstances apply to the deceased person, for example they were in receipt of a state pension or welfare benefits. This certificate is free of charge.
- **Standard Death Certificates** are issued for use by banks, building societies, insurance companies and any such organisation that requires official notification. It may be wise to buy additional copies at the time of registration as they cost more if a relative re-applies.

For more *i*nformation

- *i* Age Concern Factsheet 7 *Making your will.*

- *i* Age Concern Factsheet 14 *Dealing with someone's estate.*

- *i* Age Concern Factsheet 27 *Arranging a funeral.*

- *i* Age Concern Factsheet 22 *Legal arrangements for managing financial affairs.*

- *i* Benefits Agency booklet D49 *What to do after a death* is available from DWP offices or local probate registry offices.

- *i* Consumers Association offer a range of useful information booklets and packs about all aspects of making and dealing with wills (see page 262 for address).

- *i* Lord Chancellor's Department booklet PA2 *How to obtain probate* is available from local probate registry offices.

Conclusion

This chapter has covered a wide range of services, available from many organisations and agencies in the private, public and voluntary sectors. If you have read through the chapter briefly you may then find it useful to return to the appropriate section when the time is right, as your circumstances change.

6 How to cope with failing health

However well you care for your relative their cancer may begin to worsen. It's not always possible to make forecasts about how an illness will develop or how long each stage will last but if the person is older their health may begin to fail. The emotional side of this situation is a private matter, and you may or may not choose to ask for support, but many of the practical difficulties will be the same for all carers.

This chapter provides useful information to help you make plans for the future. It may seem difficult and even wrong to start thinking about failing health before that time has come but many families say it's less stressful to make decisions and plans about potential events whilst they are relatively calm. Talking about the forthcoming period is not morbid, it's a part of the process that helps you all come to terms with changing circumstances.

Caring for an ill person at home is a difficult undertaking and sets up a mixture of emotions. Carers experience tremendous reward coupled with extreme tiredness; they feel anxious and sad and frequently become frustrated at the inadequacies of the 'system'. Despite these hurdles it is possible to overcome the problems and most carers feel determined to provide quality care at home for as long as possible.

There are no right or wrong decisions nor are there effortless ways of dealing with the position – simply do the best you can – and make use of the help available when you feel you have reached that stage.

Short- and long-term care

New and more experienced carers continually reach stages when they need to break fresh ground – perhaps by taking on increased responsibilities and seeking additional support. The first part of this chapter helps you to assess the type of help you might need. It then guides you through the maze of information about which services are available for older and disabled people (including those with an illness) and their carers, and how they and you can access the health and social care systems. Later in the chapter, basic material is offered to help you care for your relative as their health worsens. The next chapter deals openly with caring for your relative in the terminal stages of their cancer.

Do you need help?

Margaret

'Until I talked to the cancer nurse I never realised that there were so many organisations that provide support. I would have struggled on alone whereas the help has been tremendous.'

Look at the checklist below and if you answer 'yes' to any of the questions and would like further information, you can ask for help locally. Ask at your doctor's surgery, health centre or social services office.

■ Have you just started to care for someone whose health is failing?

- Do you think the person you care for should have an assessment or re-assessment of their needs?
- Do you want to talk to someone about how you feel and what you are entitled to receive?
- Would you like to know more about respite care facilities?
- Do you feel exhausted and close to breaking point?
- Do you need help to move your relative safely – for both your sakes?
- Do you think extra equipment would help you to manage better?
- Do you feel you have received a poor quality service or support from those providing care?

Community nurse

'If you are unsure about any aspect of caring, speak to your community nurse. We know all about local services and you don't have to get the doctor to refer you.'

Although you may have been caring for a while, it is possible that you are not familiar with the full range of services. Why not find out what is available before pressure builds up and you reach crisis point. Community nurses or social workers are often thought to be a last point of call, but they can give support and advice to carers long before the crisis stage is reached. The community nurse is one of the key people for accessing other services.

The assessment process and how it can help you and your relative is described in greater detail below. It's the entry point to all types of care and is open to anyone who feels they are in need of a support service. Getting extra help does not mean that you have failed or that you are receiving charity. Families can be surprised and overwhelmed by the speed of change and deterioration of their relative. It is not wrong to make enquiries that show you are anticipating future need.

Being informed

Teresa, carers' support worker

'Take a pen and paper with you to make notes when you visit the surgery or any other professional worker. Take your time – although GPs and nurses are busy people they would not wish you to misunderstand because you are feeling frightened and anxious.'

The time may come when your caring situation changes and being informed is a major factor in maintaining control and dealing with difficult issues. Knowing what might be offered, even if you are a bit hazy, will make a basic starting point when you seek additional support. Don't try to remember everything you are told but do try to make a note of the key headings that services fall under; for example, your rights as a carer, domestic help, where you can obtain equipment. If your relative is terminally ill, help and support will be available immediately. Gathering information now could help your peace of mind and save time later when your energies will be needed elsewhere. Set up an information folder and keep a notebook if it will help organise your affairs.

Lorna, general practitioner

'The surgery is often the first place to ask for help. Keep "knocking on the door" if you feel frustrated about getting an answer – you sometimes need to make your GP understand what you want. GPs should be a signpost to other services and if you need a home visit make this clear.'

Local support services

Support for you as a carer and for your relative is available locally from a number of sources run by statutory, private and voluntary organisations. Most of these services will be accessed via the NHS or the social services departments, and your relative will be assessed as requiring 'nursing' care or 'personal' care. There may seem to be little difference in practical terms, and in reality the services try to work very closely together; however, it does make a difference to the way need for care is assessed and how care is paid for.

Changes in care provision have resulted in a National Service Framework which sets out new standards of care for older people, whether they are being cared for at home, in a care home or in hospital. There are numerous new procedures (and promises) governed by this Framework, including a one-stop assessment process for health and social care, and new legislation that will help to ease the financial burden of long term residential care. It is not possible to outline all of the procedures here so carers are advised to ask for a fuller explanation, from the appropriate authority, when making a decision about care needs.

Charges

Charges for care homes vary according to the type of care being provided. From October 2001, registered nursing care is free in England and Wales in nursing homes paid for by the NHS. In Scotland personal care is free from July 2002, in addition to nursing care. If State financial help is not required, private homes are available without undergoing an assessment; however, even if your relative is willing to meet the full fees it is possible and advisable to ask for an assessment from social services to help you choose the right sort of home and ensure that all the options are clear. Up-to-date information can be obtained from social services customer relations department or similar office in the local authority; look for the telephone number under 'Social Services' ('Social Work' in Scotland) or the Primary Care Trust.

Social services departments can charge recipients of services (but rarely carers) for many services they provide depending on personal circumstances. If a person requests services or accommodation, the local authority has a legal duty to carry out an assessment, using a set of eligibility criteria, to find out if, and at what level, care might be needed (see page 179); and to pay for meeting any necessary care costs, at the agreed level, after a means-test. A means-test is an assessment of a person's financial circumstances.

After a needs assessment is completed, the cost of any care services offered to your relative will be explained before a care plan is agreed. The rates that are charged for care services are set nationally by Government. The needs assessment and the financial assessment are undertaken separately and the results should have no bearing on each other.

For more *i*nformation

i Age Concern Factsheet 10 *Local authority charging procedures for residential and nursing home care.*

Social services

Angela, carer's support worker

'Carers are bombarded with information when they are desperate and least able to listen calmly. It's much better to take in small pieces of advice when it's most needed rather than try and remember everything at once.'

Local social services departments are the main agencies for co-ordinating community care services for older people: this book is primarily about cancer, so although for some families such information will be helpful, not all people with cancer will require direct services from a social services department. In all areas, close liaison takes place between community nurses and social workers and care will be shared when necessary.

Social services assessments, care plans and eligibility criteria

> **Carers UK**
>
> 'When carers have an assessment they get more services.'

> **Angela, carers' support worker**
>
> 'Unfortunately, services are reduced when budgets are tight. Carers must ask for a proper assessment, this is a right.'

Social services departments are responsible for providing a wide range of home, residential and day care services. These are provided direct through their own home care service, or purchased for your relative from voluntary or commercial organisations (sometimes called the independent sector). Unfortunately, demand for these services is heavy and most departments have limited financial resources so they apply strict eligibility criteria (tests) to decide which services to provide.

The first stage is an **assessment** that is intended to gather basic information about the situation and the care needs. It will take place in appropriate surroundings and time will be taken to answer your questions; however, it may happen that certain details are discussed by telephone to establish the urgency of the situation. At the end of the assessment the care needs of your relative are clearly defined and, if no further help and advice is needed, an agreement is reached with your relative (provided they are mentally capable) and you about what those care needs are. For the purpose of assessment these fall into five basic categories:

- physical safety, for example, if the person has regular falls;
- physical disability, for example mobility, sight or hearing problems;

179

- mental health, for example dementia or severe depression leading to neglect;
- loss of independent living skills, for example becoming unable to cook, wash or dress themselves;
- social needs, for example the person is very isolated and lonely.

The assessor then decides the **level of need** from **low** to **very high risk**.

Once it is decided that a person is eligible to receive services, discussions take place between everyone immediately involved to devise a care plan that best suits the needs of the family. The eligibility criteria continue to apply if your relative is already receiving services. The needs of both of you will be **re-assessed** by means of a **review** and services may change as a result of this process. Again, everyone immediately concerned will be fully involved and informed of any decisions about future care. If you do not agree with the result of the assessment, you may appeal against it via the social services complaints procedure (a social worker or care manager will advise you about the process). Social services departments will investigate any complaint seriously and will suggest that you obtain independent advice. The local Citizens Advice Bureau may be able to advise you.

Home care (social services)

Help for adults with day to day living in their own homes includes:

- personal care (such as washing, toileting, going to bed);
- practical help (such as housework or shopping) although this type of care is most likely to be provided by a separate agency;
- help for carers who may be partners, relatives or friends (such as respite care);
- advice and equipment from an occupational therapist (such as commode, bed raisers);
- help for people with specialist needs from specialist staff (such as those with hearing or sight loss, or physical disabilities).

Care assistants give personal care such as washing and toileting and do basic treatments; they are not trained nurses so do not undertake elaborate nursing procedures.

From July 2002 the way charges are made for home care in Scotland will differ slightly to that in England and Wales. Guidelines giving the appropriate charging structures will be available locally.

Health care services (NHS)

Services from the NHS for people with health care needs includes the provision of general and specialist care, loan of equipment, rehabilitation, respite health care and continuing NHS care – ie care that the NHS pays for in full. The main decisions about which health services will be provided for people locally are taken by Primary Care Trusts, which also commission services from other NHS Trusts and the independent sector to complement their own provision. You can get information about health services from your GP surgery and NHS Direct (see page 158). NHS and social services staff should work closely with your GP to maintain community care.

Local health services tend to fall into three categories:

- **acute health care,** given at NHS hospital trusts that offer specialist tests and treatments through inpatient and outpatient services;
- **community health care,** provided by NHS Primary Care Trusts that offer day-to-day care from a range of services, including community nursing, physiotherapy, occupational therapy and chiropody;
- **tertiary health care,** provided by care homes.

Eligibility criteria for continuing NHS health care

Each NHS Trust sets its eligibility criteria for these services based on national guidelines. They must be published and should be available from the local NHS body. Your relative's health care needs will be assessed against these criteria. Some older patients with cancer may have longer-term care needs than younger patients. The 'eligibility' assessment process will be broached sensitively for cancer patients. An NHS patient receiving treatment in hospital and requiring services after discharge, will be assessed before leaving hospital. If long-term, hospital-based care is not needed, social services and NHS professionals will work together to prepare a care plan (a set of services) to be provided at home or in a residential or nursing home. The care given to each patient is overseen by one senior person who will work with a small team of staff to ensure consistent care. The name given to this key person may vary from area to area but it is designed to fulfil the same purpose – the role of care 'manager'.

The views and wishes of the person and their family should be taken into account whatever healthcare is offered. If you do not agree with the decision to discharge your relative from hospital you can ask an independent review panel to look at the decision. The community health council (known as the health council in Scotland) or PALS (Patients' Advocacy and Liaison Services) can help you if you are unsure how to proceed. (PALS are new organisations which will become available on NHS sites and will help to signpost people through the health system.)

Home care (NHS)

The Community Nursing Service operates throughout the country providing nursing treatment and care for people who remain at home. Community nurses are based at GP surgeries and health centres; patients are usually referred by their GP but anyone can contact a community nurse direct. If a care plan has already been set up following hospital discharge the community nurse will call automatically. But if your relative has not been discharged recently and you feel you need help and advice, you may telephone for an assessment. Don't wait until you are desperate, particularly if your relative has become incontinent. Community nurses are a great source of local information about resources and can put you in touch with other services and arrange equipment and items, such as incontinence pads. Ask for a telephone number at your surgery or leave a message for the nurse.

Jean

'I felt so relieved when the community nurses came to us. They turned my husband at regular hours and helped me sort out how to give the right dosage for the pain killers.'

For more *i*nformation

i Age Concern Factsheet 32 *Disability and ageing: your rights to social services.*

i Age Concern Factsheet 37 *Hospital discharge arrangements, and NHS continuing health care services.*

i Age Concern Factsheet 20 *NHS Continuing care, free nursing care and intermediate care.*

i NHS Direct is a 24-hour information and helpline available in England (details on page 158).

Pharmacists (chemists) and prescriptions

Pharmacists provide a number of services to the community and are a valuable source of information about medicines, 'over-the-counter' treatments (which don't need a prescription) and minor health problems. Pharmacists will advise you to speak to your GP if they feel there is a need for medical treatment. Before you speak to a pharmacist, make a list of all medication being taken by your relative so that he or she can be sure that drugs will not interact with each other.

In particular a pharmacist is responsible for the making up of prescriptions for medicines or certain medical aids. You may take a prescription to any pharmacy but, for people living in rural areas, a dispensing service is available at surgeries and health centres if the nearest pharmacist/chemist shop is more than one mile away; ask about the availability of this service if you are unsure. There is normally a charge for prescriptions, but certain groups of people qualify for free medication; for example, people on income support; people over retirement age; and people with certain illnesses.

Having cancer does not automatically mean that people are exempt.

Pharmacists can help in other ways, such as supplying and/or filling a 'Dossit' box to help someone take the correct drug dose at the correct time of day and putting medicines in non-child-proof containers if people have difficulty opening the caps.

Cancer patients may need drugs that are not routinely stocked by pharmacies and so need to be ordered. If you speak with your local pharmacist they may be able to keep appropriate supplies in stock for your needs.

Pre-payment certificates are available to help spread the cost for people who need regular medication but do not qualify for free prescriptions. Enquire about these or any other pharmacy-related details at your local chemist shop or GP surgery.

Voluntary services

There is a wide range of voluntary organisations that provide services, self-help and support to carers at national and regional levels. Some voluntary organisations only provide services that are broadly targeted, for example advice and information available from Citizens Advice Bureaux; whilst others offer help with specific diseases such as cancer. Services provided by the voluntary sector may carry charges to cover costs.

Many of these organisations are directly contracted by the NHS and social services to provide care locally. The services are professionally managed by well trained staff; day centres for cancer patients, transport schemes and meals on wheels are good examples. National charities dealing with cancer are most likely to offer support through telephone helplines, newsletters and self-help advice.

No two areas will offer identical services, so you will have to find out what is available in your area. The two main sign-posting organisations for local voluntary sector services can be found in the telephone directory under Council for Voluntary Services

(CVS) and Volunteer Bureau (or contact the National Association of Councils for Voluntary Service or Volunteer Development England: addresses on pages 269 and 274).

Specialist cancer agencies

There are many organisations that work directly with and for people with cancer – too many to cover fully here. The larger charities offer materials and advice covering all aspects of cancer treatments and some provide direct 'hands-on' care; the smaller charities tend to offer a specialist service. Many charities also fund and undertake and/or support research into cancer. For contact details of the main charities, see the 'For more information' section on pages 89–90. Ask at the GP surgery to find out what is available in your local area. The full range of services, spread across several organisations, is very varied and may include:

- written literature, such as leaflets, fact sheets, books, newsletters;
- audio and visual tapes for people with impaired senses, and to provide clear information for all patients and carers;
- Internet access to web-site material;
- helpline services that enable patients and carers to speak to trained nurses or counsellors;
- residential homes/hospices providing accommodation and medical and nursing care for cancer patients (see page 186 for more details of hospice care);
- 24-hour community nursing care for patients in their own homes;
- access to urgent welfare items where there is a time delay or absence in statutory provision;
- research institutes carrying out research work into cancer;
- training programmes for doctors and nurses to improve the care and treatment of cancer patients and to help professional workers be better informed so that they can promote a greater understanding among the public.

The key charities are CancerBACUP, Marie Curie Cancer Care and Macmillan Cancer Relief, all of which provide additional information. Contact their national offices (see 'Useful addresses' starting on page 258) for direct information or details of what facilities are available at regional centres.

Hospice care

Hospices are available in most areas throughout the UK, provided by a combination of independent charities and NHS services. They work in close partnership, with shared facilities, to provide the best possible care appropriate to need. Patients can receive hospice-type care at a range of places; the building may not be called a 'hospice' or especially built as such, but the treatment offered will be similar. As an example, Marie Curie Cancer Care has ten centres providing skilled medical and nursing care for cancer patients.

The main services provided at hospices cover:

- In-patient care for:
    - expert pain and symptom control;
    - rehabilitation and convalescent care;
    - respite care where patients can enter the hospice for short-term treatment and return home when their condition improves;
    - terminal care.
- Palliative day care.
- Community support through specialist palliative care nurses, including a home sitting-service.
- Access to an inter-professional team of experts in palliative medicine, specialist nurses, social workers, chaplains, occupational therapists and physiotherapists.
- 'Hospice at Home'.

Hospice staff are specially trained to work with people suffering from cancer (and certain other diseases for which hospice-type care is suitable). They can advise on pain and symptom control, and give emotional and spiritual support to patients, their families and friends during the difficult time surrounding the illness and bereavement. Chapter 7 covers palliative and terminal care in more detail.

Hospice care is free of charge regardless of who provides the care. A hospice endeavours to meet the needs of people from all cultures and religions and those without an acknowledged faith. Although many hospices have a Christian foundation, this will not have a bearing on any of the services offered.

Independent care providers

Help at home is available from private and voluntary agencies that offer a range of services, including personal and domestic care, respite facilities, holiday accommodation and companionship. One such organisation, Crossroads – Caring for Carers (address on page 263), has schemes in most areas of the country. Charges made by private organisations vary and may be greater than the rates charged by social services. If you wish to obtain care from an independent agency for your relative, or to top up the amount of care they receive from the local authority, ask your social worker for details or look in *Yellow Pages* or check with one of the national organisations listed in the 'For more information' section on pages 191–192.

Margaret

'As my husband's illness got worse we made a family decision about what would be the best thing to do and we all wanted to keep him at home with us. We got help from a private care agency when he needed more care.'

Residential and nursing homes

Christine

'My father already had cancer when he went into a home and he was given good care but we visited several homes before he said that he felt it was the right one for him.'

Residential and nursing homes offer permanent accommodation to people who are unable to live independently in the community. Many homes also offer respite care facilities and other temporary arrangements.

The definition and availability of care is changing under the terms of the Care Standards Act (England) 2000 and Regulations of Care (Scotland) 2001, with new procedures starting everywhere in 2002. All residential and nursing homes will be called 'care homes' with different categories of home available, depending on the types of care offered. Various combinations of care might be offered; for example:

■ homes that offer personal care only;
■ homes that offer additional nursing care;
■ homes that offer personal and nursing care, with the facility to provide medicines and medical treatments (may be called hospices);
■ homes that also cater for people with dementia and those who are terminally ill.

Your relative can purchase all their care needs from private agencies, if they are willing to pay the charge, or, in a few specific instances, if their local authority agrees to give them 'direct payments' to pay directly for the social services that have been assessed to be needed. Nursing care is free in any setting in England from October 2001, and nursing and personal care is free in Scotland, from July 2002.

When you begin caring, you and your relative may be coping well and may not wish to consider a care home as an option. However, over a period of time, if the care situation becomes stressed or your relative's health deteriorates, moving to a home may become the best or only choice open to you both. In such a situation, it's vital that everyone involved in the decision has a chance to express their feelings about seeking permanent care. If your relative is able, you should discuss with them the merits of staying at home or entering residential care, and weigh up the possible advantages and disadvantages for everyone concerned. Think about all the factors that might influence the decision:

- The benefit of increased safety and care provided by trained staff.
- Peace of mind and less stress for the carer, especially if relationships have become strained.
- Ready-made companionship – but loss of privacy and independence.
- Feelings of guilt and the loss of a close relative from the immediate family circle.
- The costs of travel and time for visiting.
- The difficulty in finding a suitable home.
- The overall cost of residential care set against charges for care at home.

However, could your relative continue to live at home or in 'extra care' housing if the level of services were increased?

Taking the discussion a stage further

It's not easy to decide which type of home to live in and the decision should not be made hurriedly. A list of addresses can be obtained from the local authority, and details can then be obtained direct from individual homes. All homes are now called 'care' homes. Residential homes (whether run by statutory bodies, voluntary organisations or the independent sector) offer living accommodation but do not provide nursing care. It could be worth considering a home that provides both residential and nursing/medical care, if you believe that because of their illness your relative might come to need more specialist care. All types of care homes make charges according to a financial assessment, unless your relative has chosen to make their own private contract with the home and pay the full fees. Even if this is the case, it is advisable to ask for an assessment from social services to ensure that you are aware of all the options.

Ask around amongst your friends and acquaintances about the care homes you are considering. Word of mouth is a useful source of information and measure of local feeling. When you and your relative are getting closer to making a decision, gather together details, draw up a shortlist and arrange to visit the homes. It's important to get a feel for the atmosphere and care provided. If possible, see if you and your relative can visit to share a meal or other activities with current residents. You might want to ask yourselves some questions to help assess what type of home would be best.

- How mobile is your relative?
- What is their current physical and mental state and are these likely to change rapidly?
- How much care is needed – round the clock cover or day-time support only?
- What type of care is needed – nursing care including medication and treatments or personal hygiene care only?
- Will special aids and equipment be needed?

Remember also the things that your relative likes to do or feels are important – being able to attend church, favourite meals, having regular visitors or playing bridge, for example.

Registration and inspection

All care homes, whether independent or statutory, are subject to standard registration and inspection procedures, carried out locally. All inspection reports must be publicly available. You can find out more about registration criteria by contacting the local registration department; contact details will be available at your social services office. Some independent agencies belong to organisations that require them to meet their own independent standards, such as those set by the United Kingdom Home Care Association (UKHCA), in addition to the national criteria set by the Care Standards Act.

Making a complaint

If you are not happy with the services you receive from any organisation (NHS, social services or voluntary agencies) you should try to resolve the situation as soon as possible by speaking to the person involved – this could be the senior nurse on duty, your care manager or home manager. If you are still not satisfied and wish to take the matter further, contact a customer relations department or equivalent (a voluntary organisation will have a management committee) and ask for details of their complaints procedure. For independent help about how to deal with a complaints procedure contact your local Citizens Advice Bureau or community health council (or its equivalent – see the local telephone directory).

For more *i*nformation

- *i* Carers Handbook Series: *Finding and paying for residential and nursing home care* by Marina Lewycka, published by Age Concern Books.

- *i* Age Concern Factsheet 6 *Finding help at home*.

- *i* Age Concern Factsheet 20 *NHS continuing care, free nursing care and intermediate care*.

- *i* Age Concern Factsheet 29 *Finding residential and nursing home accommodation*.

- *i* Age Concern Factsheet 39 *Paying for care in a residential or nursing home if you have a partner*.

- *i* Age Concern Factsheet 40 *Transfer of assets, and paying for care in a residential or nursing home*.

- *i* *Care Homes Directory*, published by HOMES Directories Ltd, Valley Court, Croydon, Royston, Hertfordshire SG6 0HE, an annual directory giving details of over 1000 nursing, residential and respite care homes.

- *i* *Directory of Hospice and Palliative Care Services*, published by the Hospice Information Service (address on page 266), is a concise guide to over 700 hospice services provided by organisations and the NHS.

- *i* Elderly Accommodation Counsel (address on page 265) provides a national register of accommodation in the voluntary and private sectors suitable for older people.

- *i* Independent Healthcare Association is a representative and lobbying organisation for private care homes (address on page 267).

- *i* Jewish Care provides a wide range of social services for the Jewish community, particularly elderly people (address on page 268).

i United Kingdom Home Care Association (address on page 273) represents the interests of home care organisations and promotes standards of care. Its UK helpline provides information on agencies working to the agreed code of practice.

i For registration and inspection units, look in the local telephone directory, or ask at your social services department or health authority.

Facilities that support home care

Respite care

Dick
'Having a break was difficult. I went to my daughter for a few days and my wife and I did miss each other but I felt ready to carry on for a bit longer.'

All carers need a break from caring, to be alone or to spend time with other family members and friends away from the caring situation. This type of break is called 'respite care' and can take many forms.

- A couple of hours to do some shopping, read a magazine or visit a friend.
- A longer period to take a week-end break or a holiday.
- Time spent at home catching up on jobs whilst your relative goes to a day centre.
- An uninterrupted night's sleep.

Breaks like these are not a luxury – they are essential for your own health and wellbeing and will help you to cope better. Your relative might also welcome a break from the usual routine. Everyone needs to 'recharge' their energy and reduce their stress load. The Government NHS Plan recognises the importance of respite care in its *Better Care – Higher Standards* Charter, which indicates that information must be available locally about 'types of breaks for carers'. Even if you feel fine at present, try not to leave it until you are desperate for a break before attempting to make arrangements. Respite care can always be organised if there is an emergency, but it's much better to have a regular time set aside that enables you to plan ahead and have something to look forward to. The effort needed to organise a break may be more than you can take on if you are at crisis point. A social worker would explain about how carers can be assessed for provision of services.

You might be doubtful about handing your relative over to someone else, even for an hour or so, but the break should be good for both of you. A social worker or district nurse can help you make arrangements or you can contact the national agencies listed below. Try to involve your relative in making the arrangements, if at all possible. For example, if there is more than one option, your relative might want to make the choice.

- **British Nursing Association** provides care assistants, home helps and qualified nurses to care for people in their own homes. A wide range of services are offered including convalescent care, night care, personal care, shopping, companionship and respite care. The organisation caters for every level of need from occasional visits to live-in care. Look in the telephone directory for a local number or contact BNA at the address on page 261.
- **Crossroads care schemes** are the local schemes forming part of a national network set up to provide practical help and support to older and disabled people and their carers. Each situation is assessed individually with the trained care attendant taking over the role of the family carer. Using the Crossroads care scheme will give you an opportunity for a respite break at a time of your choosing; care is given 365 days of the year. Look in the telephone directory for a local number or contact Crossroads – Caring for Carers at the address on page 263.

Charges are usually made for respite care; each organisation will give you details relating to your relative's circumstances. If regular respite care is part of your relative's care from social services, ask what charges, if any, there might be. People who meet their health authority's criteria for NHS respite health care may have this provided (free of charge) in a hospital or hospice.

Day care

> **Sylvia**
>
> 'The ambulance came once a week to take Derek to the Macmillan day centre. He didn't mind going because he realised that I could go out and see a friend or have my hair cut. The social worker set it up for us.'

Day care for your relative is another way for you to have time to yourself, and for your relative to enjoy other activities and different company. All local authorities and many voluntary organisations provide day care facilities at non-specialist day centres offering support to carers and older people. In many larger towns there are day care centres offering specialist facilities to cancer patients, run by cancer charities. A range of social activities and care needs are covered. Lunch is always provided and your relative may be able to receive chiropody, hair dressing, complementary therapies, a bath if this is difficult at home, or sit quietly and doze. Some services operate in a purpose-built day centre whilst others share accommodation in community centres, residential homes and hospices. The staff are trained professional workers with additional volunteer help in many centres. For more details ask your social worker or district nurse.

Laundry services

> **Nan**
>
> 'The district nurse said that my mother was eligible for incontinence pads and the boxes arrived at the door. The pads made such a difference because I had less washing and she slept better because she stopped worrying about wetting the bed.'

If your relative is incontinent, excellent help can be found in most areas through the Continence Advisory Service. Ask at your GP surgery for details. A district nurse or continence advisor will make an assessment. Incontinence has many causes, and it may be possible to improve the symptoms considerably with treatment.

For people who have heavy urine and soiling problems, incontinence pads are available and it may be possible to make use of a home collection laundry service. Facilities vary around the country. Incontinence supplies are free from the NHS

For more *i*nformation

i Age Concern Factsheet 23 *Help with incontinence*.

Meals on wheels

A meals service is provided for many older or disabled people in all areas. It is run by the Women's Royal Voluntary Service, or other local organisations, and these reasonably-priced meals are delivered either hot daily or as a pre-packed frozen service at regular intervals. Referral is via a healthcare professional or the social services department.

Extra equipment

Carers nursing someone at home encounter greater difficulties as the person becomes less mobile. Immobility for people suffering from a cancer-related illness tends to develop gradually as their health and strength fails – unlike the abruptness of paralysis immediately following a stroke – so for you and your relative each stage can be assessed regularly and you can adjust to whatever degree of movement remains. Aids and equipment to help with moving and handling patients are used frequently by professional carers nowadays as part of Health and Safety regulations. Many useful pieces of equipment can be hired or loaned free of charge from social services, NHS trusts and voluntary organisations.

- **Wheelchair:** this is essential for mobility inside and outside the house, especially if breathing is difficult and the effort required to walk even short distances causes unnecessary isolation.
- **Urine bottle/bedpan:** nowadays many people prefer to purchase these items from a pharmacist/chemist shop, but bedpans can be borrowed or hired if required.
- **Commode:** this piece of 'furniture' is necessary in the later stages of an illness but can be useful if your relative needs to use the toilet during the night.
- **Sliding sheets:** made of a slippery nylon fabric, the two surfaces slide easily when placed together to move a person in any direction on chairs, beds and car seats.
- **Moving aids (hand held):** these firm, flat plastic supports can be placed under the thighs or the back of an individual and held by two people to make movement in a bed or chair easier. Alternatively, a banana-shaped board can be placed between a chair and the bed (or wheelchair) to slide the person across so that they do not have to be raised into a standing position. Using aids such as these puts less strain on frail limbs and shoulder joints – for both the patient and their carers.
- **Mechanical hoist:** these operate by electric or hydraulic power and are used mainly in nursing homes by professional carers for people who are very difficult to move. Hoists can also be recommended for use in the home, after assessment.
- **Bed and chair raisers:** these look like heavy-duty, plastic flowerpots and are excellent for raising furniture by several inches to ease the strain of bending and moving.
- **Special mattresses:** several types are available to help protect vulnerable pressure points when a person becomes chair- or bed-ridden.
- **Pillow support or back rest:** several types are available.
- **Handrails and ramps:** these can be positioned at various places, such as the bathroom and at the entrance to the house.
- **Bath aids:** aids range from basic non-slip mats to mechanical lifts.

- **Adapted crockery and cutlery:** for general eating and drinking, or for kitchen use if your relative enjoys helping with the cooking or wants to make a hot drink.
- **Two-way 'listening' system, mobile telephone, answering machine or entryphone:** all these offer a means of communication without the need to rush or climb stairs unnecessarily.
- **Personal alarms:** see 'Emergency help systems' on page 151.

Dick

'The commode made such a difference. It had wheels so I pushed it right over the toilet seat (without the pot), so there was no need to struggle trying to lift my wife along the landing.'

In all areas of the country, your first point of call for loan information is through a community nurse or an occupational therapist (OT). An assessment of your relative's need will be arranged. Occupational therapists work towards restoring and maintaining levels of independence and reducing the impact of illness. They may be based with social services or the NHS depending whether your relative has been referred to them because of a health or a social need. Ask the community nurse or your doctor to make a referral for a home visit if you are unsure which agency to approach. Equipment supplied by the NHS is lent free of charge. Unfortunately, waiting lists for certain pieces of equipment are long in many areas.

For more *i*nformation

- *i* The Disabled Living Foundation offers advice on aids and equipment (address on page 264).
- *i* Disabled Living Centres Council (address on page 264) can tell you the centre nearest you, where you can see and try out aids and equipment.

i Local branches of the British Red Cross or St John Ambulance give advice and arrange the hire or loan of equipment – look in the telephone directory for a contact number or ask the community nurse for a referral.

i Many pharmacist/chemist shops sell aids and small pieces of equipment or keep catalogues for mail order.

i Care and Repair England provides advice and practical help to older and disabled people and those on low incomes, to help them improve their home conditions. Charges are made, but these can be set against a grant if one is provided (address on page 262).

Conclusion

The decision whether to look after your relative at home or arrange care in a nursing home or hospice will be based on a number of factors. The wishes of the person concerned; your ability to give quality care; the support that other family members can give; and the type and amount of care that is needed should all be taken into account. It's not an easy decision and cannot be taken lightly. Caring for someone else is a time-consuming and strenuous job that draws heavily on the personal resources of the main carer. This task is almost impossible to undertake single-handed and relies on the support of the professional services as well as family and friends. If the care is long term it can put a strain on relationships and stretch finances.

Whatever your initial decision may be, it is important that you review this from time to time and accept that no carer can ever make a promise that is binding forever.

The next chapter will cover the care required by your relative as their cancer progresses – palliative care, pain control and facing the time when terminal care is needed.

7 Palliative care, pain control and terminal care

Sadly, the time may come when you have to face the news that your relative's cancer has returned or that it can no longer be treated. This stage in the illness may re-open a whole raft of feelings that have been suppressed while things were going well. If this is the case for you, why not telephone one of the cancer organisation helplines listed on pages 89–90 and talk to a counsellor about your feelings. As has been stated many times in this book, specialist help will be available to support you through the difficult times – none more so than now, when your relative is approaching their death.

This chapter concentrates on what happens during the relatively short period when your relative requires terminal care. The time-lapse from first diagnosis and treatment through to this stage will be different for everyone, but the information needs of most carers remain the same. Many families wish to assist with the terminal care of their relative and want to be well informed about such things as freedom from pain, how to deal with emotions and how to provide practical, sympathetic nursing care.

If you are the main carer, it is probable that you are feeling afraid; that you are unsure what to expect; and that you need support yourself. It is also probable that you are the solid rock that others rely upon. Family members may turn to you as the central figure at times of crisis, and, although you may feel comfortable taking this role, you must also be wary of taking onto your shoulders too great an emotional load passed on by everyone else. Wherever possible keep the family channels of communication open because, as your relative enters the terminal stages of their cancer, you may need to draw upon your family's patience and help as you focus all your mental and physical energy on the person who is ill.

In the final stages your relative may begin to understand that they are close to death; some people embrace this stage peacefully whilst others are less accepting. It may be the case that you and your relative approach this time differently. This chapter will help you to accept that death brings a mixture of emotions and to recognise when death is near.

Palliative care

'Palliative' is a term used to describe the treatment given to patients when cure is no longer the aim of treatment, and the emphasis of care is on relieving suffering and maintaining quality of life. Palliative medicine is a distinct speciality offering an active, total approach to treatment of a patient with regard to their physical, social, psychological and spiritual needs. Palliative care includes family support and bereavement services.

During the course of the illness certain procedures used to ease discomfort may have been described as palliative treatment. For example, low doses of radiotherapy, minor surgery and/or chemotherapy are all used to relieve pressure on nerves and other organs. However, in the last stages of terminal illness the only palliative treatments given are those which make the final weeks of life as comfortable as possible.

Wherever your relative is nursed – at home or in a hospice – they and you can expect to receive high quality care and services derived from your rights to:

- comfort;
- non-discriminatory behaviour;
- respect and dignity;
- adequate and appropriate therapies, treatments and support;
- accurate and comprehensible information.

If for any reason you feel that your relative, or you as the carer, are not receiving the standard of care that you desire then approach the appropriate manager and explain your concerns. The local Community Health Council (or its replacement service – see your local telephone directory) can offer you advice.

Controlling pain

Elaine, a doctor

'Approximately one in three cancer patients experience little or no related pain, and as pain is felt more severely by some people than others, we treat each person as an individual.'

Fear of pain affects everyone, especially when a diagnosis of cancer has been made. In the early stages your relative (hopefully) will have been reassured that if pain occurs, from the developing cancer or as a side effect of treatment, it can be controlled effectively with modern drugs.

Reasons for pain

Pain occurs because:

- the tumour is pressing on a nerve or a nearby organ. Occasionally 'referred' pain is felt away from the cancer site

201

because the nerves carry the pain some distance;
■ an infection may be developing at the site of the cancer (or elsewhere) with increased pressure from fluid or pus;
■ scar damage may have occurred to tissues following surgery;
■ radiotherapy treatment may cause discomfort;
■ the cancer may have spread to a secondary site; for example, aching in a limb may be caused by a secondary bone cancer (metastases). Some people describe this as a 'dull' ache.

Early reporting

If your relative is in discomfort it is important to tell this to a member of the medical team, wherever they are currently receiving treatment – at the outpatient clinic, the GP surgery, a general hospital or a hospice. It's advisable to talk about this at an early stage so that the level of pain can be assessed, treated and monitored for change.

Elaine, a doctor

'There is no reason at all for your relative to suffer in silence, because they are unsure about how much pain they should bear or they believe that pain with cancer is inevitable. If any part of the body hurts then tell a doctor or nurse and let them decide on the best course of action. It may not be possible to eliminate the cause but all pain can be helped.'

One of the reasons for reporting pain promptly is that reassurances can often be given that dispel anxiety. Not all pain is connected with the cancer, there may be other causes that need attention; for example, muscle pain from a strain or discomfort from arthritis. Neither does the amount of pain necessarily indicate how severe the cancer is or that it is getting worse; however, it can be a good measure.

Before your relative asks for advice, you could help them to define the pain as concisely as possible, perhaps by jotting down a few notes. The clearer the information given to the nurse or doctor, the easier it will be to decide on treatment. The main points to clarify are:

■ which area of the body is affected;
■ whether the pain moves around or is always in the same spot;
■ whether it gets worse or better at certain times of the day;
■ what it feels like – a dull ache, a sharp continuous pain or an intermittent stabbing sensation;
■ whether it resembles other pain felt in the past – toothache, or headache, a pulled muscle or like having a baby;
■ how bad it is – rate it on a scale of one to five to which future pain can be compared;
■ whether it can be improved or ignored by using certain tactics – taking a rest or a walk, warming or cooling the body area, concentrating on something other than the pain;
■ whether the pain interferes with other day-to-day activities, such as sleeping, eating or hobbies.

Dealing with the pain

How to deal with the pain can be approached at two levels: firstly, at a self-help level with home management, complementary thera-pies and over-the-counter remedies relieving the symptoms of mild discomfort; and secondly, using medication that needs to be pre-scribed. There are a number of more complex non-drug methods of treating pain such as palliative radiotherapy. The answer often lies in being flexible and finding out which treatment methods work well, singly or in combination, and using the information to manage the situation. The nurse or doctor can help you and your relative draw up a list of treatments that complement each other to eliminate the danger of over-dosing on a mixture of prescribed and over-the-counter medicines.

Self-help and non-drug treatments

Many techniques can go a long way towards relieving mild to mod-erate pain. Try a combination of the methods.

Self-help treatments

Complementary therapies Several well-tried treatments can be used to ease aches and pains; for example, acupuncture and acupressure, aromatherapy and massage are very straightforward methods to try at home. Hypnotherapy can help to relieve the symptoms of pain, induced by a trained hypnotherapist or as a self-help method. Contact the National College of Hypnosis and Psychotherapy (address on page 270) for a list of qualified hypnotherapists or ask for information at the GP surgery or cancer centre.

Counselling Talking to a trained counsellor about anxieties and fears surrounding pain may help reduce stress levels and improve your relative's feelings about the future. Ask a cancer nurse how to arrange counselling or contact a national cancer charity helpline (see pages 258–274 for addresses and telephone numbers). Talking to family members is also very beneficial and a relative or friend may be able to recommend a local, private counsellor. The British Association for Counselling and Psychotherapy publishes a directory of counsellors in the UK (address on page 260).

Distraction Concentrating on strategies that help take the mind off the symptoms can reduce the tiring effect of pain. Use well-tested examples, such as listening to music or a talking tape, reading and watching television. It's also worth trying alternative methods such as visualisation and relaxation techniques (see Chapter 8) that are easy to learn at home.

Position Make sure the body is positioned comfortably so that muscles and scar tissue are not being stretched beyond their natural spot. Change position regularly to ease pressure and relax muscles. Use aids such as sheepskins and pillows to give support. Straighten out bed covers and change bed linen often. Try a different chair or mattress if well-used furniture has become less comfortable. (See page 196 for a list of other aids.)

Temperature Changing the external body temperature can have a very comforting effect. Use whichever method feels appropriate, for example a rubber hot water bottle; a gel-filled container that can be warmed in a microwave oven or cooled in a freezer; make up an ice-pack with crushed cubes or use a bag of peas. Be aware of safety as well as comfort and always use a protective covering between the appliance and bare skin. Sometimes alternating hot and cold brings effective relief and for overall sensation try a warm or cool bath.

Tens machine This piece of equipment can be used to stimulate nerves reaching the brain to encourage the body to produce its own pain killers, natural chemicals called endorphins. The mild, electrical stimulation is not unpleasant and works in a similar way to acupressure (see page 87). The small, battery-operated machine can be carried easily in a pocket. The equipment is readily obtainable; ask for information at the GP surgery or cancer centre or from a physiotherapist.

Specialist non-drug treatments

Nerve blocks This technique aims to block the pain 'messages' that travel along the nerve pathways. Several methods are used; for example, long-acting local anaesthetics injected into the site; cryotherapy (freezing technique); or heat therapy (radiofrequency thermo-coagulation technique). These treatments can only be accessed via the medical services.

Radiotherapy This treatment is used to treat pain in bones and some other sites. Low doses only are necessary to achieve very effective results. The therapy takes time to start working so other pain killers will need to be taken until the benefits are felt. It may then be possible to reduce the dosage of stronger medication. This therapy can only be accessed through your relative's medical team.

Medication used to control pain

The information given here is intended only as a brief outline of the main drugs used to control pain so that you and your relative understand why the medication is so important and what effects it can have.

It can be confusing for a non-medical person when the words 'drug' and 'medicine' are used to describe any form of medication but they mean the same thing. Although there seem to be many drugs used to treat pain there are, in fact, only a few main groups, described below. This apparent abundance of drugs is because:

■ any one drug may be available in several forms;
■ the doctor may try several drugs to find the combination which gives the best results with the least side effects;
■ different manufacturers make the same basic drug in different preparations. Think of medicine like coffee on a supermarket shelf – the trade names and the packaging are different but the granules are the same!

Sean, a doctor

'Taking responsibility for their relative's drug regime is a job that many carers have to undertake. If you don't understand about any treatment you can ask the doctor, the cancer nurse or the pharmacist at the chemist shop.'

Professional people will give you considerable support but you will also have to take responsibility for certain aspects of your relative's care. Be aware of your relative's mental state – if there is any chance that they might be confused about which drugs to take or how much, do not leave any form of medication out for them to take later. The correct dosage must be supervised. If your relative is able to take their drugs safely but has difficulty opening containers, ask a pharmacist for details of specially designed tablet boxes with separate compartments that you can load with a day's supply. If you are concerned about getting the timing and doses right, because your relative is taking several drugs, it might help to write out a chart as a memory aid.

The following basic rules apply to any medication:

■ Follow the instructions given on the label.
■ Never stop using a prescribed drug without taking medical advice

■ Take the dose regularly, at the stated times, to achieve the intended result.

■ Never take more than the prescribed dose – if the pain persists or becomes worse, seek advice.

■ Store all medicines in a secure, locked place away from children and any person who may not handle the drugs safely.

How do drugs get into the system?

There are three main ways that drugs enter the body: the most common route is through the mouth. However, some drugs work better by being injected into the blood stream and occasionally they are absorbed via the skin. Most pain-controlling drugs are taken orally in tablet or liquid form but other methods are used, for example skin plasters, suppositories, injections, intravenous drips and automatic syringe drivers. It is unlikely that all of the ways described below will be prescribed for your relative.

■ **Anal suppositories** are inserted into the back passage for slow absorption. Morphine may be given this way.

■ **Intramuscular injections** are given deep into a muscle, usually the buttock or thigh.

■ **Intravenous injections** involve inserting a liquid drug into a vein, rapidly by syringe or slowly by a drip. Chemotherapy drugs are given this way.

■ **Implanted lines,** for example Hickman or central lines, are designed to be left in for a period of time. They consist of a length of plastic tubing inserted under the skin and fed into a large vein in the chest. Drugs are injected through the protruding end.

■ **Oral route** is used for tablets, capsules or liquid, from mild analgesics such as Panadol to a quick-acting opium-based syrup.

■ **Spinal cord route** is used for severe pain. A small catheter is inserted into the spinal cord by an anaesthetist and attached to a reservoir of the drug. A top-up dose of drug is injected whenever it is required.

■ **Self-adhesives patches** giving a slow absorption of the drug are sometimes used to relieve severe pain. Fentanyl, a strong pain-killer used as an alternative to morphine, is given this way.

■ **Subcutaneous route** is made just under the surface of the skin, for a single injection or for longer-term action whereby a tiny needle is placed permanently under the skin to inject a regular supply of the drug using an automatic syringe operated by a battery or clockwork pump, carried unobtrusively in clothing. Relatives who feel confident enough may be taught how to change the syringe daily.

Common pain relievers

The main drugs used to relieve pain for cancer come from several sources; common examples, morphine and codeine, are derived from opium. There are many drug combinations open to the doctor, so the types and quantities can be prescribed according to current need. Pain-killers may cause drowsiness so care must be taken. It is important to read the instructions as it may not be safe to drive or take alcoholic drinks. Pain-killing medication comes in three strengths, providing mild, moderate and powerful relief.

■ **Mild pain-killers,** such as paracetamol, aspirin and ibruprofen, are all available as prescription drugs from the hospital or a GP or over the counter from a pharmacy. Some drugs have more than one function, for example, ibruprofen and aspirin also help to reduce inflammation. **Never buy products for your relative straight from the shelf without taking advice.** A trained pharmacist will be able to advise on appropriate medication. Be sure to tell the pharmacist about all other medication and treatment your relative is receiving, as a pharmacist is trained to be aware of drug interaction and which drugs may or may not be suitable.

■ **Moderate pain-killers,** such as codeine, are often prescribed in combination form with paracetamol to give the best results, for example *co-codamol* or *coproxamol*. Many drugs that have the same effect will be marketed under different trade names (see above). Some moderate pain-killing drugs can only be obtained by prescription supplied by a doctor, others with lower doses of codeine or its equivalent can be bought over the counter.

■ **Strong pain-killers,** such as morphine, are given to control severe pain. These drugs can only be obtained by a medical prescription as they are subject to very tight, legal controls. The dose of morphine is carefully adjusted to ensure adequate pain relief and to minimise any unwanted side effects such as drowsiness. A common way of starting morphine treatment is with an instant-release preparation that starts to work after about half an hour, the dose being repeated every four hours and more frequently if pain persists (often with a 'double dose' at night to avoid waking the patient). Once a suitable dose has been established the doctor is likely to prescribe a slow-release version that acts over a period of 12 to 24 hours. Morphine does have a few, unwanted side effects in some people. Constipation is nearly always a problem and the doctor will be aware of this and may suggest that laxatives are taken at the same time. If nausea is a problem, medication can be taken to help ease the feeling; this usually settles. A dry mouth is a minor side effect that can be improved by drinking plenty of fluids, sucking sweets, pineapple chunks or chewing gum. Drowsiness or confusion can be troublesome but usually settles once the dose has remained the same for a few days. If morphine causes too many unpleasant side effects the doctor will prescribe an alternative medication that is just as effective.

■ **Other medication:** other drugs may be prescribed to work together with pain killers. The most commonly used ones are: non-steroidal anti-inflammatory drugs for pain in bones; steroids to help reduce swelling and for certain types of pain associated with damage to nerves; anti-depressants, anti-convulsants and sedative drugs. All of these drugs can have unwanted side effects and your relative may be advised to take them with a meal and/or take an anti-acid type medication.

Becoming addicted

Freda

'My mother kept refusing the pain killers because she was afraid of what she had heard about getting hooked. She was less anxious when the doctor explained that such fears are common, but that addiction does not happen when people take strong drugs for pain.'

The level of dose relates directly to the level of pain – it does not relate to the severity of cancer. The dose of any pain-killing drug is carefully worked out and monitored to achieve the desired effect, which is to control the pain until the next dose is due. The doctor will start a patient off on a low to medium dose and increase it according to need. Different people have different pain thresholds. If the dose is not sufficient to control the pain, tell the doctor – it may need to be increased or supplemented with a second drug. The reason why drug addicts become addicted and crave for larger doses is because they are seeking greater drug-induced pleasure; they are not using the drug to ease pain. A degree of physical dependence does occur with patients taking morphine for pain and the medication should not be stopped abruptly. If the cause of the pain is removed (for example, if the pain was caused by a secondary cancer in a bone and the pain has been improved with palliative radiotherapy) then the dose of morphine can be reduced slowly and discontinued – your doctor will tell you how to do this.

For more *i*nformation

i CancerBACUP booklet *Feeling better – controlling pain and other symptoms* (see page 261 for address).

Terminal care

Susan

'Somehow I felt calmer because my husband died in our own home. I know that not everyone can manage care at home but I had lots of help from the community nurses and my family.'

Ron

'My wife was moved to a hospice just before she died. I couldn't care for her as well as the nurses because she needed constant attention. She was looked after so well I felt we had made the decision that was right for us.'

Caring at home for a relative with a terminal illness is a time of great emotional and physical strain. It is not easy to make predictions about how long the final stages of an illness will last or how much care a person may need. People whose health is deteriorating have good and bad days and may remain on a plateau for quite a while, supported by medication and nursing care, before they finally slip into unconsciousness. If you are continuing to nurse your relative at home in the terminal stages of their illness, you will be offered support from the local community nursing team. Specialist palliative care community nurses will be available for advice and support, and work closely with the community nurse from the NHS trust. Arrangements vary around the country: some specialist palliative care community nurses are part of a hospice team, some are Macmillan-trained nurses working from a hospital-based support team or a community team; Marie Curie community nurses provide hands-on nursing care at home, and are available across the country. The nurses assigned to your relative will assess how much care is needed and will visit several times a day if necessary. In some areas there are special flexible services that provide help to settle

211

patients down at night and give pain-killing and sedative drugs, and all-night nursing services to sit with very ill people. Your relative's doctor and community nurse will make the necessary arrangements.

Returning home from hospital or a hospice

If your relative has been ill for some time, you will already have some understanding of the system; Chapter 6 outlined what help and support is available, from which services. Nevertheless, services constantly change so, however well you think you know the system, it might be sensible to have a chat with a nurse and/or hospital-based social worker a day or so before your relative is due to be discharged, to update your knowledge and check which care services are still in place. Facilities that were previously supplied may have been changed or withdrawn whilst your relative has been in a hospital or hospice. Your relative's GP should automatically be informed about the discharge but you may wish to make contact with the surgery yourself.

If you are new to caring, the immediate practical support necessary for your relative's wellbeing will be set up before they leave hospital. A social worker and/or discharge nurse will explain the procedures to you. Whatever is arranged for the early days, remember that you and your relative are entitled to an assessment (see page 179). The situation can be reviewed as circumstances alter and services may be increased or adjusted according to the results of the assessments.

As well as speaking to members of the medical team, discuss the proposed care with your relative so that you are both clear and happy about the arrangements for the immediate future. You are entering a shared process of 'taking care of' and 'being cared for'. By sharing hopes and concerns with each other (however ill your relative may be) you are each having a say in the care plan. The level and amount to which your relative realistically becomes involved may depend on how frail they are. The key point is that they are offered the opportunity to take decisions and have a say in their own care – a very empowering position and one to which they have a right. It may be helpful to include other family members in the discussions about the caring process. Even if you are the person who takes charge of the practical care, there are lots of other jobs that will need doing and sharing the caring load spreads the responsibilities.

Practical arrangements, such as preparing a suitable room, doing a big supermarket shop and starting to draw in family and friends as part of your support network can all take place before your relative leaves the hospital or hospice. A number of issues may need to be discussed thoroughly before discharge day; for example, decisions about where your relative returns to live; whether they are able to get upstairs to sleep; and, if it is your partner, do you continue with the same sleeping arrangements? The answers to these questions may depend on several factors determined by their ability to care for themselves; available household space and personal choice. Whichever decisions you make initially, be flexible and adjust arrangements as necessary.

Care over the final days

Being able to take special care of a relative in their remaining days is very important to families, particularly if you are looking after your relative at home, not least because it enables you to retain a sense of control. Of course, professional people will be around to help and advise you, but they may not be at hand exactly when you want to ask a particular question. The main care will be provided by a team of professional people, community nurses (who will take responsibility for all nursing procedures) and care assistants who provide personal care. The doctor, community nurse or social worker will organise these services on your behalf. You will be asked to take care of your relative between their visits and maybe assist them with some procedures that need several pairs of hands. The following list is a guide to the needs of a sick person.

- **Personal hygiene:** bathing, washing, nail cutting, hair washing, mouth care, moisturising, attention to pressure areas and changing bed linen.

213

- **Drinking:** offer fluids regularly when your relative is awake to quench their thirst and help to keep their mouth moist. Buy a specially-shaped feeding cup, baby feeder or flexi-straws from a chemist shop as it's easier to control the flow of liquid from a smaller opening. Flavoured, crushed ice is good as a mouth refresher, as is fresh pineapple.
- **Eating:** very sick people are rarely interested in food. Offer small light portions that provide nourishment without bulk. Do not be concerned if the food is refused; take the plate away without pressure to eat. Keep a supply of ice cream, yoghurt and custard handy as these foods are easy to swallow.
- **Moving and turning:** regular movement is important to help ease discomfort and avoid sore pressure areas. You will be advised about how to move your relative safely.
- **Medication** (including pain control): when giving any drug (particularly strong pain killers) take care over safe storage, accurate doses and correctly spaced timing. If your relative has difficulty taking a drug in one form ask the doctor if there is an alternative method which can be tried. Keep a note of how well the drugs are controlling symptoms and whether there are any adverse effects.
- **Night care:** the community nursing team will tell you about specialised nursing services provided by charities such as Marie Curie nurses.
- **Toileting and dealing with incontinence:** your relative may lose control of their bladder and/or bowels if they are semi-conscious. This can be very distressing so ask for a supply of incontinence pads or whether a urinary catheter can be fitted.
- **Wound dressings and clinical procedures:** all nursing-type care is covered by the community nursing team.

Dealing with the final hours

When your relative is approaching death

When a person is terminally ill with cancer, the time will come when they are close to dying. Being with a loved one who dies at home can be a very tranquil experience, knowing that you have done all that you can to help them die peacefully in their own surroundings. However, it is not too late, even if you have been coping well at home, to ask that your relative be moved to a hospice. If you or they would prefer this the GP will organise the transfer arrangements and the staff will try to do everything possible to make you and your family feel comfortable.

Fiona, cancer nurse

'As the time approaches when your relative is dying you may be concerned about how you will cope. Try to bring yourself to talk to a nurse as we can advise you about what steps you need to take. Ask the staff to let you help with the care, so that you can remain involved and continue to do the best for your relative.'

Dying with dignity

There are many ways in which family, friends and medical staff can help to ensure that the expected death of a person is approached with dignity. It is probable that in the terminal stages of any illness the person (if they are conscious) will be aware of their deterioration and the changes that are taking place in their body. Some people recognise the inevitability of death and become peaceful, whilst others continue to struggle and are less accepting. Sometimes the ill person and family members are at different stages of acceptance; in this case it may help to talk to each other or to someone who is less involved. If the ill person has accepted that death is close, relatives must respect this feeling and not beg them to hang on to life. We have certain obligations towards a dying person. In

215

practical terms, these focus on their right to be kept clean, warm, comfortable and free of pain. Perhaps less easy to understand is any need for emotional and spiritual fulfilment, often because a person close to death is unable to express in words what they actually feel or desire. Sitting quietly by their bedside may be enough.

Fiona, cancer nurse

'Being close by is very important. If you are able, talk to your relative, ask them about their wishes and give them an opportunity to talk and feel at peace. If your relative is unable to respond they may still be able to hear you. But be careful about discussing sensitive matters within their hearing.'

Over the final days, if appropriate, your relative may wish to spend time doing some of the following things:

- Talking with the people they hold dear, including friends and family, to reminisce about past times; to tell them about their love, which may include saying sorry for past disagreements. To be reassured that someone will talk to younger children.
- Talking about their fears of death and what might lie ahead, perhaps with a non-family member so that privacy is maintained.
- To be reassured that they are not being a nuisance, particularly if they lose control of bodily functions.
- To know that all their affairs have been put in order, including the wish to make or amend a will, and to feel that they will have left sufficient means for a spouse or other dependant to live in reasonable comfort.
- To have someone sitting with them at the time of death and to receive any spiritual or religious rites that are part of their cultural belief.
- To have helped plan their funeral service by choosing hymns, psalms and readings.
- To know that a final resting place for their body or ashes has been agreed and that any requests to be buried or cremated in special clothes or wearing a piece of jewellery will be respected.

Common fears

Jill, cancer nurse

'Even though I have worked in a hospice for years it is not easy to comfort a dying person as our society has few words to use in a situation about which we have no direct experience. I suggest that relatives listen with sympathy and offer words of gentle support that allow the dying person to talk about their fears.'

Most people hold some fears about dying, especially when they are terminally ill. They can often sense that life is drawing to a close and may experience deep anxiety and even panic at the uncertainty ahead. Apprehension about dying is a natural fear that should never be suppressed or dismissed as foolish by healthy people. Until faced with the reality of death few people ever think about its implications for themselves or how they will react. The things that people fear most are:

- pain;
- the process of dying;
- the unknown place following death;
- losing their faith;
- losing control, especially increasing dependence on others and incontinence;
- being a burden to others and what carers might think;
- possible judgement after death, depending on their religious beliefs;
- dying in an unpleasant manner;
- dying alone;
- being buried or cremated alive.

Recognising that death is imminent

Timing matters greatly and many people find it easier to cope with the thought of the forthcoming period if they have some idea when to expect the death.

> ## *Jill, cancer nurse*
>
> 'Many relatives ask professional carers "How long will he live?" Clearly, there can be no definite and precise answer to this question but it may be possible for nurses to give some idea of time scale. For example, if someone is already unconscious the final descent leading to death is unlikely to be drawn out. This period may last days but could more easily be expressed in hours. We try to give a gentle warning at this stage to help prepare you for the approaching death and support you to accept the certainty of the situation.'

At the time of death you may wish to sit by the bedside and hold your relative. When a person is dying their breathing often sounds noisy and their body may become restless. These changes are part of the process of death, they are not signs of distress. A dying person usually slips into a coma and is not aware of these actions. Gradually breathing slows down and stops. If you wish to check that death has occurred you can also feel for a pulse at the wrist. Make a note of the time of death. Afterwards it is all right to sit quietly with your relative for a while and adjust your thoughts.

After a while you must inform someone of the death. If you are in a hospice the staff will be close by and a nurse may be with you at the time of death. If you are at home, you or another family member must telephone your relative's doctor so that they can confirm the death before issuing the Medical Certificate of Cause of Death. The GP or a member of the hospice staff will explain what to do next (see pages 170–172).

Laying out your relative

You may like to wash your relative and dress them in clean clothes or help a nurse to do this. The hospice staff or undertaker will do this job if you would prefer not to, and you can stay with the body, or not, as you choose. If your relative has died at home you can call the undertaker, at any time of the day or night.

Fiona, cancer nurse

Fiona, cancer nurse

'People behave in different ways immediately after the death of a loved person. How you actually feel and behave may be different to how you imagine you will respond – there are no right or wrong feelings at this time.'

The factors that make a difference about how you feel tend to reflect:

- **The age at which the death occurred:** a younger person rather than an older person.
- **The timing of the death:** an expected death rather than a sudden death.
- **The relationship and bonding between the people concerned:** an older parent losing a child or a young person losing a sibling.
- **Whether the bereaved person was present at the death:** people are often very thankful that they were there until the end.
- **The existence of unresolved disagreements prior to the death:** use the opportunity to express love for each other.
- **Support from family and friends:** a listening ear or a meal cooked are supportive acts that need no thanks.
- **The influence of spiritual or cultural beliefs:** ritual and custom can be great ways to relieve stress and fill empty moments.
- **Whether blame or resentment is present (justified or not):** it is not uncommon for bereaved people to seek a scapegoat upon which to direct anger.

For more *i*nformation

- *i* CancerBACUP booklet: *Coping at home: caring for someone with advanced cancer* (address on page 261).
- *i* Carers Handbook Series: *Caring for someone who is dying* by Penny Mares, published by Age Concern Books (see page 277).

ℹ *Directory of Hospice and Palliative Care Services in the United Kingdom and the Republic of Ireland*, published by the Hospice Information Service (see page 266 for address).

Conclusion

This chapter may be difficult to read as your relative enters the final phase of their life. If they are being nursed in a hospice the staff will have taken care of some of the immediate practical arrangements. If your relative remains at home, dealing with basic household tasks can sometimes take your mind away from the hurt. In the days immediately following the death people often feel numb and shocked – these are natural feelings.

Sometimes people also feel a sense of alarm or frenzy at the thought of all the things to do after someone has died – but they don't know where to start. Return to Chapter 5 for information about how to register a death.

8 Managing stress

Caring for someone who is unwell is stressful for many reasons: the overriding sadness of a potentially life-threatening illness; anxieties about the future; and the extra pressures of trying to manage your own life alongside caring for your relative all contribute towards mental and physical fatigue. It's no wonder most carers say that feelings of tension never go away.

This chapter describes the main elements of stress and helps you focus on your personal problems. How you deal with a difficult situation depends on lots of factors. Your personality type, how well you feel in control and how much energy you have in reserve, all play their part in your ability to cope.

We all need a few strategies to draw on when we feel at the end of our tether. This chapter looks at ways to build up your personal strengths and develop some support systems and offers a selection of coping skills to use when you need to remain calm and reduce the tension. Relaxing your muscles or enjoying an aromatherapy massage can work wonders when your are feeling pressured and over-tired.

The advice given in this chapter is intended to help you make use of self-help techniques that will support you while dealing with everyday problems, some of which might stem from your caring role; it is acknowledged that your relative's illness is likely to be at the root of your distress and that no amount of stress-reducing strategies will ever take away that hurt.

What is stress?

Rita

'I have never felt so tense in my life before. I feel like a piece of stretched elastic – I couldn't give another inch.'

The word 'stress' is very popular nowadays and is commonly used to describe the way we feel when pressure is intense. It's not a medical problem but a combination of symptoms produced when our physical, mental and emotional systems go into overdrive. Everyone's body reacts to stress in the same physical way, whatever the cause or size of the problem. Unfortunately, though, some people's mental processes seem to get more upset when faced by difficult situations. This stronger reaction to stress is often produced by a combination of factors – their emotional state at the time, what their personality type is and how well they have learned to cope in the past – rather than the extent of the problem.

High stress levels for carers are likely to stem from:

- loneliness and isolation;
- shortage of time;
- uncertainty about the future;
- difficult relationships and pressures from other people;
- feeling that life is getting out of control;
- lack of sleep;
- feeling under-valued and over-worked;
- lack of knowledge.

Primitive feelings

Claire

'I developed such horrendous headaches and they were always stress-related.'

Coping with day-to-day stress is normal because a small amount of pressure can improve performance. It keeps your brain stimulated and helps you concentrate and deal with challenging situations. For example, many actors regard a bit of stress as essential: it adds sparkle to their performance and keeps them alert. But when the pressure becomes too great the reaction can be unpleasant. As tension builds up your body produces high levels of adrenaline hormone to prepare itself for action in the same way as a primitive caveman. This reaction, known as the 'fight or flight' mechanism, enabled him to respond swiftly to danger. Nowadays, though, unlike our ancestors, this type of 'escape' is rarely necessary, so instead of using up the energy generated to deal with the hazard it remains in your system, keeping it in a continual state of tension. While adrenaline levels are high, you probably feel as if you are living on the edge of a crisis so it takes little additional worry to make you feel very anxious. The tension can become so intense that you may feel as if you are about to explode and you can no longer handle all of the demands being made of you. If you 'listen' to your body it is telling you that it feels extremely distressed.

Peter

'My wife was in hospital and I had to keep working as well as visiting her. We ran a small garden centre and it was coming up to our busy time of the year. The thought of doing the accounts filled me with dread.'

223

Valerie

'When my mother was ill I had my father-in-law to see to as well. My husband and I would have given anything for an offer of help from someone.'

Warning signs

Rita

'When my mother lost her spectacles yet again I nearly exploded. Why couldn't she remember where she had dropped them? I'd had a dreadful day at work, my back was aching and I wanted a bit of space.'

Claire

'When my boss started piling on the pressure I felt sick with anxiety and angry with her; she knew my husband was ill, why couldn't she be more thoughtful?'

The signs and symptoms that indicate that you might be feeling over-stressed are triggered by a combination of physical and emotional reactions. Check the list below and note the symptoms that trouble you regularly. If you are bothered by more than a few, the time is right to consider some solutions before your own health begins to suffer.

- Headaches
- Feeling tired and listless
- Difficulty in sleeping at either end of the night
- Palpitations and rapid pulse rate
- Indigestion/heart burn
- Breathing problems (faster and shallower)

- Aching joints
- Over- or under-eating
- Skin problems
- Increased urine output and nervous diarrhoea
- Numbness and pins and needles in limbs
- Poor concentration and difficulty making decisions
- Feeling unhappy and depressed
- Feeling angry, frustrated and helpless
- Feeling irritable and tearful
- Feeling anxious and fearful
- Lost sense of humour

Where do all the stresses come from?

Charles

'My wife tried to protect me even though she was ill, but knowing that made me feel worse. I felt that I had to be strong for both of us.'

Valerie

'I nearly collapsed the day the washing machine leaked. Problems were building up with no time to think. I mopped the floor and cried with exhaustion – how could life be that cruel?'

It is difficult to define stress clearly because it feels as if it comes from two directions, both external and internal. The confusion arises when we talk about stress as a cause of problems (pressures from people or situations) or as an effect (a response from inside our bodies, such as a tension headache). Both internal and external stresses affect our moods and the physical ability to cope. Unfortunately, not all sources of stress are within our control, and problems can rarely be packaged neatly into distinct 'causes'.

225

Mostly we manage to keep the troubles isolated and give our bodies sufficient rest before dealing with the next set of problems.

Psychologists refer to these sources of stress as 'life events' and they include major upheavals like retirement, moving home, changing job, an accident and illness but also lesser events such as Christmas or going on holiday. They aren't particularly special or rare and they aren't necessarily unpleasant, just things that happen to all of us all of the time. However, if a string of events happen too close together, pressure builds up to uncomfortable levels and it only takes one small problem to bring everything to a head. The important point to note is that it is the accumulation of both major and minor events that happen close together that creates the worse effect, rather than merely the severity of the events.

Stress triggers

Peter

'It was raining, the car wouldn't start and I still had all the shopping to do. I tried to ignore the light-headed feeling from too little sleep and no lunch.'

If built-up tension is already at critical level, it won't take much to tip you over the edge. Do the following 'nerve janglers' seem familiar?

- Tiredness caused by insufficient sleep due to frequent interruptions in the night, or altered sleep patterns such as waking early.
- Prolonged pain perhaps from aching joints or the continual physical strain of moving an ill person.
- Fragile emotions stemming from anger, sadness or anxiety.
- Frustration and pressures created by people or places – relatives, hospital appointments, shopping in crowded supermarkets.
- Discomfort caused by lack of fresh air, too much noise or feeling too hot or too cold.

- Depressing weather; some people are adversely affected by too little sunlight and long dark evenings.
- Sensitive digestive system; too much alcohol, caffeine in tea and coffee or refined sugar can all exacerbate stress.
- Craving for a cigarette because anxiety levels are high. Long spells waiting in a hospital environment make smoking less easy. Stress is the reason many people give for continuing to smoke.
- Uncertainty about the future and possible financial worries.
- Impatient personality – some people tend to be quicker to react than others.

Two personal stories

The stories of **Jenny** and **Brigid** are typical examples of how stress builds up into distress.

Jenny's story

'My husband and I had just set up our own business when my father was diagnosed with a cancer. The next few months were a nightmare. I felt that my time and my loyalties were divided, causing a great deal of anxiety. I went to hospital with him while he had diagnostic tests and chemotherapy and then rushed back to do the paperwork and telephone clients. I still felt worried after he settled back at home because I didn't know how well he was taking care of himself. I couldn't sleep because I was uncertain about the future and began to feel unwell with quite a lot of physical and emotional symptoms – bad headaches, extreme tiredness, poor appetite and feelings of panic. The final straw came when our house was burgled. I felt completely shattered and didn't know where to turn for help.'

Brigid's story

'I had been taking care of my mother for six months following her operation for cancer and I was beginning to feel that I couldn't carry on. Besides looking after her, the rest of my life threw up the usual problems. I had to teach my class at the secondary school, mark pupils' work in the evenings and support my daughter who was taking her final exams at college. I was very tempted to start smoking again even though I had given up several years ago. The situation came to a head one day when I exploded at my class, treating a minor event like a major disaster. When the situation had calmed down I was left feeling drained, trembling and confused at the strength of my own emotions. Fortunately, a colleague at school persuaded me I needed to ask for help. I went to my GP, who arranged for me to see a qualified counsellor within the practice. It helped enormously to talk to someone who listened without passing judgement.'

Brigid and Jenny had each gone through a difficult period in a short space of time with a run of problems adding to their stress load. Each story illustrates the pattern that can lead to a build-up of pressure:

- a series of stressful events close together;
- little control over the individual situations;
- burdens from other people;
- little time for personal relaxation.

Brigid was lucky to have had a caring colleague who recognised the signs of stress and suggested she seek help. She found a safety valve by talking to a counsellor. Be aware of early warning signs and learn how to recognise your own body signals so that you can help yourself before you reach discomfort level. However, there are no magic formulas – stress management, like any other skill, needs to be learned and practised.

Getting the balance right

The key to managing stress is getting the balancing act right between tension and relaxation – like a juggler, if you get too many plates in the air at once they all come crashing down. Caring brings extra responsibilities and you may be the main person your relative relies on, so balancing your own needs against theirs may be hard to achieve. Unfortunately, you are the one most likely to end up with too much stress and too little time for relaxation. Tension and anxiety can't be switched off to order but this does not mean they should be ignored. There are ways to ease the pressure and give your body a rest, and stress is easier to bear if you understand and accept where the problems are coming from.

Brigid

'I have learned that I am not superhuman so I think about what jobs need tackling and I divide them into those that are urgent and those that can wait. It's amazing how my mind clears when I have sorted out the priorities.'

Peter

'When I stop and reflect on how I coped, I know that I tried to keep each part of my life separate. While I was visiting my wife in hospital I put work to the back of my mind and while I was at work I did what I had to do and delegated some of the load to others.'

Stress diary

Writing a stress diary can help to sort out where some of the pressures are coming from. It may seem like yet another task, but a few minutes spent now may save you from sleepless hours later. Start the process by making a list of all the things that have bothered you in the last week. Next jot down by the side of each problem how you felt at the time – angry, anxious, irritable, etc. Now circle the things that you chose to do, willingly – they may have been difficult, but if you accept their importance you are less likely to be upset by the effort. Look at the remainder of the problems on your list and ask yourself if they could be the cause of your increased

229

anxiety. Are they stemming from external pressure over which you have little control? The reason why many people get angry and upset about some situations and not others is often linked to their feelings about choice. Can you cross out anything off your list to ease the pressure?

Pauline

'My husband is ill and needs care. I want to look after him at home for as long as I am able, however difficult. We are very close and I believe he should be in his own home with the animals and familiar things around.'

Because Pauline has made a personal decision to care for her husband she feels calm about the outcome.

Mental stimulation

Roger

'I wanted to be at home to take care of my wife when her cancer was diagnosed so the decision to take early retirement was mine, but I did miss the company of the office. While my wife goes to the cancer day centre one day a week I always spend that following my own hobbies. I play golf or go to the bridge club – whatever I fancy.'

Stress doesn't always arise from over-activity. It's also possible to feel frustrated and unsettled if you are bored, isolated at home, or doing the same repetitive jobs day after day. It is unrealistic to believe you can exercise control over every aspect of your life, but at least try to give yourself relative peace between the stormy bits. For example, if there is pressure at home, don't take on extra responsibilities outside of the house and use respite time to do something relaxing rather than a strenuous activity.

230

Helping yourself

By now you've probably got a clearer picture about the main causes of your stress and feel ready to make some changes that will
help you to cope. Start the process by asking yourself how you
dealt with difficult situations in the past and what lessons you
learned from that process. Then think about what is different this
time round and what steps might be needed to help you get along.
Remember that problems are rarely solved in isolation so think
about who (or what) you could turn to for support. Finally, accept
that not all problems can be 'solved'. The illness of your relative
may not disappear but you can try to deal with it in the best way
possible.

Finding ways to cope with pressure

No one ever cured their stress overnight so don't rush into hasty
decisions. Look at each problem separately with four courses of
action in mind:

One Is it necessary to change the situation? This course may call
for major action, such as moving your relative into a nursing home
(or hospice). Making a decision of this nature will be extremely
upsetting so don't attempt to make it alone. But if you are finding
it very difficult to cope, it could be the right longer-term solution.

Two Can you improve your ability to deal with the situation? Your
stress levels might fall quite dramatically if you ease some of the
pressure on yourself and your time. A practical solution, such as
getting help with the housework, could be the answer.

Three Do you need to change your perception of the situation?
Ask yourself if the problem is as bad as you think it is (the problem that's worrying you right now – not the cancer) and try to turn
some of the threats into challenges. Positive 'self-talk' works well
here; tell yourself that you have dealt with difficult situations
before and that you have ample reserves of inner strength.

Four Would changing your routine help? Doing things through habit is easy, especially if you are feeling upset, but your routine may be increasing your stress. If you are rushing around frantically, slow down so that your actions become calmer. This gives your brain a less stressed message. Cut down on the amount of coffee and tea you drink; the caffeine they contain stimulates the nervous system causing irritability and insomnia. Change any routines which are particularly tiring; for example, avoid shopping at the supermarket at busy times.

Pauline

'I spend a small amount of money getting the grass cut to ease the burden. My husband used to do all the practical jobs, but I was grateful when my neighbour did some decorating and we use hospital transport to get to the clinic.'

Charles

'My daughter lives nearby and she sits down with me each evening and we talk over what jobs need doing the next day. I can sleep better if I have sorted out in my mind what to do before the nurse arrives.'

Personal resources

Brigid

'My mother's cancer isn't going to go away and I have to continue working. So after my outburst I felt concerned about my state of mind. I must have a bit of space for myself or I wouldn't be able to carry on. I went to see a counsellor and she helped me draw up a list of my main strengths and encouraged me to draw on the support of people I trust. It was very reassuring to think about all of my personal resources. I value my:

- firm relationships with my husband, children, family and friends;
- good physical health;
- positive mental attitude (usually!) – I feel confident and enjoy my job;
- sense of humour;
- financial security;
- spiritual support;
- non-dependence on smoking, alcohol or drugs.

The counsellor also encouraged me to think about where I could help myself further. Together we agreed I could improve my ability to cope by:

- finding more time for myself and having a relaxing hobby;
- learning to say "no" sometimes;
- cutting back on some of the household jobs that are not a high priority.'

Like Brigid, you can also identify your strengths and think about where you feel vulnerable. Then talk to someone you trust about what steps you could take to improve the areas where you feel insecure, at least to the point where you feel less anxious.

Jenny

'I've learned not to keep it all bottled up, and meet with friends occasionally. We rarely talk about my worries, but I know I can, when I need to, and it helps.'

Brigid

'It never crossed my mind that I could ask for counselling. I had always thought that counselling was for people who couldn't deal with life. How wrong I was – four sessions with a trained counsellor made all the difference to how I coped.'

Finding support

Any support is valuable when you are feeling under pressure, especially the undemanding type that comes from family and friends. Asking for help is not a sign of weakness; it's more an awareness that problems can seldom be solved alone. You may need to make the first move and ask for a listening ear, as friends and relatives may be reluctant to interfere unless they are invited. Once you have given the signal inviting help, you should discuss with the other person how this can be achieved without upsetting your relationship. It's important to agree a few basic rules at the beginning, because the last thing you want is someone marching in and taking over. For example, the person you talk to must respect your need for confidentiality; you may become emotional and let off a 'bit of steam' and you must feel free to ignore their advice without them taking offence.

If talking to a friend or relative is not the best course for you because you would find this uncomfortable or there isn't a suitable person, other options are available.

- Specialist palliative care services are able to offer stress counselling, psychological and spiritual support.
- Many cancer centres now also offer psychological or counselling support to carers, and stress management.
- Self-help and carers' groups run by social services, health trusts or at a carers' centre.
- Private counsellors – ask at your GP practice or the Citizens Advice Bureau for a list of professional counsellors who are trained and registered.
- Religious leaders.
- Telephone helplines such as those operated by most cancer charities (see pages 89–90) or CarersLine run by Carers UK (see page 262).
- The Samaritans is a national 24-hour helpline staffed by trained counsellors who offer emotional support to people who are feeling isolated and in despair. You will find the telephone number in your telephone directory.

Decreasing the tension

Eva

'The doctor suggested a group at the carers' centre. I was unsure at first, but I found that although it didn't change the fact that my husband is ill, I coped better with it all. We always ended with a relaxation session and I went home feeling calm and supported.'

If your body is already feeling tired and strained, any movements that increase muscular tension are an extra drain on your energy reserves so its worth being as relaxed as possible. Ask a friend to observe your general posture or catch sight of yourself in the mirror or a shop window. Look out for uncomfortable positions and bad habits:

- head thrusting forward or bent down with your chin hard on your chest;
- shoulders hunched and rounded;
- arms held tightly across your chest or stiffly by your sides with hands clenched;
- legs crossed over and twined together;
- restless habits such as tapping fingers and feet, or hair twisting;
- nail biting and teeth clenching.

Better breathing

Breathing is an unconscious action that you rarely think about, but over the years you may have developed poor breathing habits without realising their significance. Irregular breathing patterns such as hyperventilation or overbreathing can increase anxiety levels. When your body is calm, breathing is slow, regular and deep, but when anxiety levels are high the opposite happens, breathing becomes fast, irregular and shallow, creating feelings of panic. Breathing is normally controlled by the involuntary nervous system but it's possible to take control of the process and calm the system down when pressure begins to rise. People who learn to breath calmly when they are feeling tense soon notice an improvement in their anxiety state. The following guidelines will help remedy overbreathing and generally reduce tension:

■ As soon as anxiety levels begin to rise, quietly tell yourself to 'calm down'. This sends a positive message to the brain.

■ Slow down all your movements, because rushing around increases agitation and your body responds by producing more adrenaline to deal with the 'threat'.

■ Calm your breathing deliberately and keep an even rhythm with a slight pause between the in and out breaths; imagine a candle in front of your face which gently flickers as you breathe out.

■ Practise calm breathing at different times during the day so that you are aware of the feeling of taking control; it's much easier to recognise the correct pattern when you are not over-anxious.

Jenny

'I found that once I had learned to control my breathing I became more relaxed generally. The uptight feeling went away and I felt less agitated.'

Learning to relax

Deep relaxation is an excellent way to restore energy and boost your spirit but it does need time and space. Merely telling yourself to relax rarely works, especially if you are feeling overwrought. Relaxation is easy to learn but it does require practice; it may take several sessions to get it right and it helps if you understand how the technique works. It's all about fooling the system and giving out positive signals that your body is at ease. Relaxed muscles and slow, quiet breathing send calming messages to the brain that turns off the false reaction to danger. When there are no threats your body rests and restores itself ready for the next burst of energy.

Whole-body relaxation

This is the most common form of relaxation and produces pleasant results quickly. The technique works if you create the right conditions and allow sufficient time – about 20 minutes for a whole-body session. Eventually, you can cut down on the time and recreate the stress-free feeling anywhere as you improve your skill. If you would like to learn to relax with a teacher ask at your GP surgery; many stress counsellors run individual or group classes.

Step-by-step technique for use at home

1 Find a warm, quiet place and lie on a rug or sit in a well-supported chair. Use a pillow for support if it helps to make you more comfortable. Reduce outside noises if possible.

2 Wear loose clothing and remove glasses and shoes. Lie on your back with head supported, arms and legs straight and slightly apart.

3 Breathe in and out deeply for three breaths and imagine you are losing tension; then breathe normally.

4 You can close your eyes at this stage or wait until they shut naturally. (You are going to work on each major muscle group starting with the feet. As you tighten and relax the muscles, learn to recognise the difference between tension and relaxation. Hold each constriction for a few seconds and repeat each action with a short break between.)

5 Pull your feet towards your body – hold the tension – release, and feel the reduction in tension.

6 Point your toes hard away from your body and feel the tension in your calf muscles – hold – and relax.

7 Next work on your thighs by drawing your legs tightly towards you or raising them into the air – hold – drop back to a relaxed position with thighs rolled outwards.

8 Tense your buttocks by squeezing them hard together – hold – and relax.

9 Tense your abdomen in the opposite way by pushing it outwards – hold – and then let it flop.

10 Check your legs again and if you have slipped back into a tense

position, repeat from step 5. A couple of deep breaths will help at this point. Your lower body should feel heavy, warm and relaxed.

11 Now concentrate on your back. Arch your spine away from the floor or chair – hold – and let go. (**Warning:** Leave this one out if you have any back problems).

12 Now move your shoulders backwards to expand your chest – hold – and release.

13 Tense your shoulders next by raising your arms and pulling on your shoulders – hold. As you drop your arms, wriggle your shoulders up to your ears and relax with your shoulder blades touching the floor or chair.

14 Now work on your hands and lower arms by making a tight fist – hold – and relax, letting your fingers droop. As you clench your fists for the second time, raise your arms slightly off the ground and notice the tension in your forearms – hold – and release.

15 Move to the upper arms by bringing your hands across your body, close to your chest – hold – relax them to a position on the floor with palms facing upwards.

16 Relax your neck and throat by gently moving your head from side to side (not a circular movement) and then pulling your chin down to your chest – hold – and release.

17 Next clench your jaw by clamping your teeth together – hold – and let go so that your mouth is slightly open. That tension probably felt familiar as clenching teeth is a common habit.

18 Now work on your facial muscles. Press your lips together – hold – and release. Push your tongue hard to the roof of your mouth – hold – and let it drop to the floor of your mouth.

19 Move your eyes inside your closed lids to the four quarters of a circle and then let your eyelids relax.

20 Finally, relax your forehead and scalp. Frown hard and pull your forehead down – hold – and let go so that your face feels floppy.

Your whole body should now feel comfortable and free from tension. Breathe gently and let your mind wander at will. If stressful thoughts irritate you in this relaxed state, think about somewhere pleasant and, as you breathe, repeat in your mind 'peace in and pressure out'. Don't worry if you drop off to sleep at this point; eventually you will learn to relax your body without going to sleep, but use this method at night if insomnia is a problem.

Lie quietly with your eyes closed for a few minutes enjoying the warm feeling; then slowly bring yourself back to the present. Count backwards from five to one, clench your fists tightly, relax and rub your hands together. If you are lying on the floor, roll onto your side; open your eyes with your hands shielding them from the light. Stand up slowly and try to hold on to the relaxed mood when you return to action.

Getting the best from relaxation

Sharing the session with another person is pleasant. You can take turns to read the instructions or make yourselves a tape recording. Listen to music if it helps to calm your mind and ring the changes by starting at the top and working towards your feet. As you become better at 'switching off', shorten the session and create a relaxed mood by imagining your body is warm and heavy without going through all of the muscle-tightening steps. Use this short-ened version as a 'mini restorative', particularly when you are away from home in stressful situations.

For more *i*nformation

- *i* British Association for Counselling and Psychotherapy publishes a direc-tory of counsellors in the UK (address on page 260).

- *i* *Understanding Stress* booklet from the Family Doctor series, available from most chemist shops.

- *i* Music tapes: 'The Fairy Ring' and 'Silver Wings' by Mike Rowland and 'Spirit of the Rainforest' by Terry Oldfield are soothing tapes to use for relaxation, available from music shops or by catalogue from New World Music (address on page 270).

- *i* International Stress Management Association UK produces a wide range of materials to help reduce stress: leaflets, audio tapes, books and a newsletter (address on page 268).

ⓘ Royal College of Psychiatrists publishes a range of information for dealing with anxieties, phobias, depression and bereavement. Send a sae to the address on page 271.

ⓘ *Staying Sane: Managing the stress of caring* by Tanya Arroba and Lesley Bell, published by Age Concern Books (details on page 280).

Complementary treatments to help with stress

> ### Sheila
>
> 'While my husband was at his day centre my sister treated me to a weekly aromatherapy session. It was wonderful. I would never have done such a thing on my own but we went along together.'

The terms 'alternative therapy' and 'complementary therapy' are used to describe a range of treatments available from practitioners and therapists who work to treat the whole body, either alongside, or instead of, treatments offered by conventional medicine. To help make clear the differences in meaning, the following descriptions are commonly accepted.

■ **Conventional medicine** covers a range of treatments which your relative may have already received, including chemo- and radiotherapy, hormone treatment and surgery. These therapies have been widely used throughout the world for many years and have undergone expert clinical trials.

■ **Unconventional medicine** covers a number of treatments that are widely used and, on the whole, widely respected. Included in this group are homeopathy and herbal medicine. Neither type is specifically used in cancer treatment and practitioners do not claim the medications used will cure cancer but the treatments may help to reduce the symptoms caused by the cancer and the side effects of orthodox treatments.

- **Complementary therapies** are intended to be used along-side rather than to replace orthodox medicine; examples include physical treatments such as aromatherapy and reflexology and treatments that benefit the person's state of mind, such as counselling and psychotherapy. The treatments may be beneficial for yourself and your relative, as complementary therapies can help to combat tension and stress and give a welcome boost to your morale.
- **Alternative therapies** are usually held to be treatments that are given instead of conventional treatments. These therapies often involve regimens that attempt to treat the cancer direct, using non-medical methods; examples include specific diets and megavitamin therapy and treatments that try to boost the immune system. Most alternative treatments have not been subjected to clinical trials.

Many popular complementary treatments originated in the East and have been practised there for centuries. They rely on ancient knowledge linked to herbal remedies and traditional practices that are believed to stimulate the body's own healing powers; acupuncture from China and yoga from India are obvious examples. Some of the newer therapies appeal more to Western scientific minds and are used as aids to diagnosis as well as treatment. Two examples are colour therapy, that draws links between certain colours and mental harmony or stress, and iridology that examines the eyes for clues to hidden disorders.

All complementary and alternative treatments can be obtained without going to a medically trained doctor but this does not mean that an NHS or private doctor will not or cannot provide some complementary treatments; some doctors are dually trained and GPs are beginning to recommend the benefits of such therapies. Increasingly, complementary therapies are being introduced into the NHS and are available at cancer centres and GP practices, either free of charge or with a fee. Geographical location may affect your ability to find a suitable practitioner; ask at your local library or GP practice or cancer centre.

A note of caution: before using any complementary or alternative therapy with your relative, especially if they are undertaking other treatments such as chemotherapy, it is extremely important to consult with the oncologist. There are several reasons for seeking advice before starting a non-orthodox treatment: some therapies use extracts from plants that can have very powerful properties that may affect other treatments; the effort of being massaged may be too tiring for a weakened body; and some therapies use methods that have not been scientifically tested. There is some conflict of opinion between supporters of conventional medicine and supporters of alternative therapies; many doctors providing orthodox treatment are concerned that alternative therapies may be harmful. Patients sometimes reject conventional medicine and seek alternative remedies out of a false sense of hope and promises of amazing cures. There is no justifiable evidence that such cures exist and no reputable therapist would ever make such claims.

Finding a qualified therapist

Several of the therapies described in this chapter can be practised at home using basic remedies and techniques learned from a book; however, rather than spend time learning new techniques, you and your relative may prefer to receive treatment from a qualified practitioner. Some alternative therapies cannot be recommended for self-help practice and it is advisable that treatment is obtained only from a trained practitioner. Ask for details of reputable, local therapists at your GP surgery or cancer centre or contact the national organisations listed under 'For more information' on the following pages. Word of mouth can be a good form of recommendation but do make sure any therapist you visit is registered to practice with the appropriate national body.

Don't be embarrassed to ask directly about qualifications, as all trained therapists will be pleased to offer reassurance and tell you how to check. Properly trained therapists take a full medical history before prescribing and have learned about the dosage and combinations of herbs, whereas untrained people can only guess and may do harm. There are some ready-made treatments available in health shops, but before taking any over-the-counter medication, it would be wise to consult a doctor first, so as not to delay diagnosis or effective orthodox treatment. Finally, whichever alternative treatment you choose it's wise to consult a medical doctor if symptoms persist. If you use information from a book to prepare treatment materials be sure to follow the instructions carefully.

You and your relative may be sceptical about whether complementary therapies work or not, especially if they rely on less orthodox and 'unseen' methods. No therapist or practitioner of complementary therapies will ever claim to 'cure' a patient alone or to replace orthodox medicine, but they would strongly support the notion that their treatments can contribute towards a feeling of wellbeing. People who use a practitioner can expect to receive more time for treatment, a whole body approach to their problems and advice about self-help. If your relative's health is failing it's well worth considering some of these treatments as they can bring tremendous relief from distress and discomfort.

Aromatherapy

Sara, aromatherapist

'Aromatherapy may be used to bring about a deep sense of relaxation and wellbeing, reducing the negative effects of stress and anxiety.'

The ancient art of aromatherapy combines the healing properties of aromatic plant essences with massage and is an excellent therapy to try if complementary treatments are new to you and your relative (see 'A note of caution' on page 242). Its gentle methods encourage a relaxed feeling and a trained therapist will ask questions first to discover the best treatment for each individual person. The complex essential oils extracted from many plants are introduced into the body where the 'life force' of the plant's essential oil can have a beneficial effect. Therapists do not claim that the oils heal directly in the sense that a synthetic drug may effect a cure, instead it is believed that the oils encourage the body to use its own natural healing forces from within. The essential oils are absorbed through the skin and pass through the tissues to the blood stream and so travel around the body. Different oil combinations affect different parts of the body, for example, camomile can help with digestive problems.

Sara, aromatherapist

'When buying aromatherapy oils, always choose "pure essential" oils to ensure a good quality is purchased. Labels which state "fragrance" or "blend" are synthetic and are useful only as mood creators or to scent a room. There are recognised retail outlets in most high streets – try good health food, bodycare and herbalist shops and the larger supermarkets.'

Essential oils are extracted from plant essences by a special distillation process that changes their chemical composition. They are used in concentrations that are many times stronger than their original plant form and are rarely used undiluted because they are too powerful to use directly on the skin. It is important to be aware of the potency of essential oils and that their use is not advised with people who suffer from certain conditions, in particular, a history of miscarriage, haemophiliacs, advanced varicose veins and during a high temperature. Always read the instructions carefully before use or follow the advice of a therapist.

Methods for use at home

Sarah, aromatherapist

'Try a ten-minute, luxuriant aromatherapy bath, using two drops each of lavender, sandalwood and ylang-ylang pure essential oils, at the end of a day to promote a peaceful and restful night's sleep.'

The soothing oils can be used in other ways to enhance their effect:

■ **Vaporisation** creates a very pleasant effect by burning oils in special containers, so that the aroma is inhaled from the air. It is believed that the healing part of the oil is breathed into the body and passes through the membranes of the lungs into the blood system. Fill the bowl with water, add two to four drops of essential oil and place a lighted night-light candle underneath. Pottery containers and blended oils are readily available in many gift shops.

■ **Oils** blended with hand and body creams give extra benefits for skin care.

■ **Hand/foot baths** with five drops of blended oils added to the water can relax the body or ease aching joints.

■ Use in **steam inhalers** or droplets on a handkerchief to bring relief from colds and catarrh.

■ Use as **room fresheners** by mixing two drops of essential oil in a cup of cool, boiled water and spray the air using a plant sprayer; or mix a few drops of blended oil with *pot-pourri* or put a few droplets onto a cloth and lay on a radiator.

■ As an **aromatherapy massage** (which has little in common with the traditional Swedish version that is much more vigorous). Simple massage techniques, such as arm massage, can easily be learned from instructions and pictures in a book.

For more *i*nformation

To obtain a list of qualified practitioners in your area contact one of the following organisations:

i Aromatherapy Organisations Council (address on page 259).

i International Federation of Aromatherapists (address on page 267).

i International Federation of Professional Aromatherapists (address on page 267).

i Bookshops and most libraries carry a range of suitable books on aromatherapy or ask the organisations above for a list of recommended books.

Bach Flower Remedies

These Remedies are named after the medical and homeopathic trained doctor who researched the healing power of plants in the 1930s. He believed that the characteristics of disorders, whether physical or psychological, could be treated by a cure drawn from plants, sunlight, spring water and fresh air. In practice the Remedies tend to be used to treat psychological symptoms. This does not imply that the conditions are imagined, simply that they stem from whole body experiences that effect the mind as well as the body. Good examples are the conditions which cause people to feel worried, depressed, exhausted, irritable and panicky.

People have always made use of medicinal herbs, but the 38 Bach Remedies claim to use the essential energy within the plant rather than actual plant material. The healing energy is stored in a preserving liquid that can be bought in a concentrated form known as the *stock remedy*. The concentrated forms are then diluted by mixing with pure water and an alcohol preservative. It's usual to combine several concentrates together to form the required final treatment. Because the action of Bach Remedies is mild, they cannot result in unpleasant reactions or side effects and can be used with all age groups. Although orthodox medicine cannot offer a sound reason for their claimed effects, practitioners believe that, by looking at psychological symptoms, people are encouraged to review other aspects of their behaviour, lifestyle and attitudes and this self-awareness contributes towards the healing process.

Bach Remedies are available at many health shops and through trained therapists. They are intended primarily as a self-help form of treatment and it is very easy to understand and prepare the Remedies using books. The following list gives suggestions about how the Remedies can be used; to treat yourself you need to read about them in more depth:

- For exhaustion and feeling drained of energy by long-standing problems, use olive.
- For the after-effects of accident, shock, fright and grief, use star of Bethlehem.

■ For apprehension for no known reason, use aspen.

■ For tension, fear, uncontrolled and irrational thoughts, use cherry plum.

Rescue Remedy Five of the Remedies – cherry plum, clematis, impatiens, rock rose and star of Bethlehem – were combined by Dr Bach into an emergency treatment he called 'Rescue Remedy'. It can be used for a number of problems associated with shock and injury to help create a calm, soothing feeling. It can be bought as liquid or cream preparations for internal or external treatment and can be used on cuts, bites or after a traumatic experience.

For more information

i To find your nearest trained practitioner and details of publications, tapes and educational material, contact the Bach Centre (address on page 259).

i A comprehensive booklist, including *The Twelve Healers and Other Remedies* by Edward Bach, can be obtained from C W Daniel Company Ltd (address on page 263) or the Bach Centre (address on page 259).

Homeopathy

Homeopathy uses minute amounts of natural substances to enhance the body's own healing power. The practice is centuries old and is widely used as the sole form of treatment or as a complement to orthodox medicine. The name 'homeopathy' is derived from two Greek words – 'homoeos' (similar) and 'pathos' (disease). The principle is that the patient is given minute doses of a substance that, in a healthy person, would cause similar symptoms to those shown by the ill person. By creating a similar condition, the homeopathic remedy stimulates the body to heal itself. The skill lies in knowing the potency of the substances and matching these to the specific signs and symptoms described by the patient. Treatments are prescribed individually. Occasionally, symptoms may worsen but this is usually a short-term effect, an early stage of the healing process.

The remedies are prepared in a unique way by repeatedly diluting plant and mineral extracts or substances that cause sensitivity (for example house dust). Unlike herbal medicine, in which only the direct effects of plants are used, homeopathic remedies are designed to treat the whole person, not just the illness, so the person's overall physical and emotional state would be assessed. There are few diseases or conditions for which homeopathy cannot be used, although there is still the need to use orthodox medical treatments. Homeopathy cannot cure what is irreversible and if long term orthodox treatments have suppressed the body's natural powers these may take a while to regenerate.

Neil, doctor

'Practitioners are trained in homeopathic medicine and many also have a general medical qualification. Homeopathic medicine is available through the NHS but practitioners may not be located in all areas of the UK.'

For more *i*nformation

To find your nearest homeopathic practitioner contact:

- *i* British Homeopathic Association (address on page 261).
- *i* Society of Homeopaths (address on page 272).
- *i* Homeopathic Medical Association (address on page 266).
- *i* The organisations above will provide a booklist, or a bookshop or library may have books on homeopathy.

Reflexology

Peter

'I was unsure about the benefits of reflexology and about letting a therapist touch my feet as they are very sensitive. But once I got into the
course it really felt helpful and it didn't hurt.'

Reflexology also complements orthodox medicine and involves
massaging reflex areas in the body, found most commonly in the
feet and hands, that correspond to all parts of the body. Practitioners believe that healing is encouraged by applying pressure to
these points to free blockages in energy pathways. The reflex
points are laid out to form a 'map' of the body, the right and left
feet reflecting the right and left sides. A reflexologist takes a full
history from the person and uses both feet to give whole body
treatment. It's an ideal way to boost circulation.

The method has been used for several thousand years and is
described in ancient Chinese and Egyptian writings. It does not
claim to cure all problems but many conditions respond well to
reflexology, especially those related to stress – migraine, breathing
disorders and circulatory and digestive problems for example.

The practitioner will initially examine the feet for signs of the primary causes of conditions, which may originate from another
system of the body, before moving on to precise massage. This
involves applying firm pressure with the thumbs to all parts of the
feet that correspond to the body areas giving problems. These
related areas in the foot feel especially tender when massaged and
the level of tenderness indicates the degree of imbalance in the
body. The skill of the reflexologist lies in their ability to interpret
the tenderness and apply the correct pressure, bearing in mind
that some people have more sensitive feet than others. The number of treatments will vary according to the condition and the
response. Reflexology is a relaxing therapy which relies on the
healing power of touch rather than substances; at the end of each
session people usually feel very warm and contented.

For more *i*nformation

ⓘ To find your nearest practitioner contact the Association of Reflexologists (address on page 259).

ⓘ The Association of Reflexologists (above) will provide a booklist or visit a bookshop or library.

Visualisation

> ### Paul
>
> 'When my wife could no longer go out for a walk I would say to her, "let's go for a walk together over the hills" and we would shut our eyes and walk for miles in our minds. It gave us so much pleasure we could almost feel the wind.'

Visualisation is a method similar to meditation but it needs much less concentration and is easier to perform. It works well whether it's done alone or with someone else. Therapists use visualisation as a healing exercise to help lift the effects of depression and to create a positive attitude towards life-threatening illnesses; it can have powerful psychological effects. It is believed that visualisation influences the brain centres that control hormone and immune systems and helps strengthen the healing process. Using it at home is an excellent way to shut out other stressful thoughts and to mentally take yourself somewhere that induces pleasure. The technique works by creating a sense of contentment and pleasure so that the brain responds to this lack of threat by telling the systems of the body to go into 'rest' rather than 'alert' mode. The reverse will happen if you visualise an unpleasant image; you may have noticed that if you think about a difficult situation, your body immediately responds by rousing itself for action, even though the event is imagined.

As your relative becomes too frail to journey far, you can 'visit' a place that you have enjoyed in the past without too much effort. First you need to sit or lie comfortably in a quiet place. Then decide where you want to go and talk to your relative by giving them an imaginary 'guided' tour along familiar paths. Start and finish your journey using similar words to these:

'Close your eyes. Today we will visit ... It is time to bring our journey to an end and come back home. Open your eyes, gently stretch your limbs and start to think about the present.'

Other therapies

There are many other types of therapies which can be used to complement each other and orthodox medicine. You can find out more about them at your local library:

- **Chiropractic** relieves pain through joint manipulation.
- **Herbal medicine** uses the potent healing properties of plants. **Note** that these preparations must always be used with caution; like all drugs, they can have unwanted side effects.
- **Hypnotherapy** induces a trance-like state to bring about physical and mental changes.
- **Hydrotherapy** uses water treatments to purify and heal the body.
- **Osteopathy** is a manipulative therapy used widely in orthodox medicine.
- **Shiatsu** is a Japanese form of massage based on the idea that good health depends on a balanced flow of energy through specific channels in the body.
- **T'ai-chi Ch'uan** is 'meditation in motion'.

For more *i*nformation

The following organisations will give you advice and supply you with further details of specialist organisations or ask at your local library:

251

- British Holistic Medical Association (address on page 260).

- Centre for Study of Complementary Medicine (address on page 262).

- Institute of Complementary Medicine (address on page 267).

- National College of Hypnosis and Psychotherapy (address on page 270).

- National Federation of Spiritual Healers (address on page 270).

- CancerBACUP booklet *Cancer and complementary therapies* (address on page 261).

- *Reader's Digest Family Guide to Alternative Medicine*, published by Reader's Digest, available from bookshops.

Conclusion

Stress is normal in small amounts and harmful when it becomes so severe that it feels *distressing*. The warning signs are common to everyone; however, some people because of personality type or a previous unpleasant experience react to pressure more quickly than others. The key to managing stress is learning to recognise where pressures are coming from and then working towards changing the situation or accepting that some situations cannot be controlled.

When your body gives off the tell-tale signals that tension is rising, try to calm yourself by slowing your movements, breathing quietly and evenly and relaxing your muscles. Let your shoulders drop and unwind all the parts of your body that have become tense. Use your support systems and don't feel it's a weakness to ask for help or show signs of emotion. Crying or shaking are good ways to relieve tension. Some complementary treatments provide excellent ways of relieving tension and giving yourself a reward. They should always be used alongside orthodox medicine, never as substitutes for conventional treatment.

Glossary

AIDS (acquired immune deficiency syndrome): the late stages of the infection HIV (see below) which includes a rare pneumonia and skin cancer (see Kaposi's sarcoma below).

Antibodies: a specific form of blood protein produced in the lymphoid tissue (see below) that are able to counteract the effects of bacteria and toxins.

Barium (sulphate): heavy white substance used in x-ray diagnosis. The barium forms a dense shadow that light cannot penetrate (opaque) giving an outline of the shape and size of the cavity which is being photographed.

Benign: the word generally means not harmful; it is commonly used to describe a non-cancerous tumour.

Biopsy: the removal and examination of living tissue from the body, usually for examination under a microscope to assist in the diagnosis of cancer.

Blast cells: immature blood cells (erythroblasts) that develop in the bone marrow. The number of underdeveloped cells in a blood sample is counted to give an indication whether leukaemia may be present.

Carcinogen: a substance which plays a part in the development of cancer. They are found in the environment and may be man-made or natural matter.

Carcinoma: a malignant growth of epithelial tissue which covers surfaces on the inside and outside of the body. It is the commonest type of cancer.

Corpuscle: a small body or cell found in blood or connective tissue.

CT (computed tomography) scan: is an x-ray examination technique which shows structures in a particular plane (section) as clearly-focused images. Used mainly in the investigation, diagnosis and management of cancer, the technique is especially valuable in showing where a tumour may be altering the shape of an organ.

Cytotoxic: any substance that destroys cells. 'Cytotoxic' drug treatment, known as 'chemotherapy', is commonly used to kill cancerous cells. 'Toxic' means 'poisonous'.

Electrolytes: substances in which minute parts (molecules) have been split into separate, electrically-charged particles, when dissolved in fluid. Mineral salts, which occur naturally in the blood, are a common example. In medicine, a test to check the concentration of electrolytes present in the blood gives valuable clues to the diagnosis of different diseases. For example, levels will be lower due to fluid loss because of diarrhoea or vomiting or more concentrated if the kidneys are not excreting efficiently causing fluids to be retained.

Fallopian tubes: tubes which are attached (one on each side) to the womb at one end, with the other end lying close to the ovaries to catch the ejected eggs.

Geiger counter: instrument for detecting and measuring radioactivity.

Genes: the biological units of hereditary which pass on characteristics from each parent.

Haemoglobin: the colouring material which produces the red colour of blood. The 'globin' part is a protein and the 'haemin' part is an iron-containing pigment. The main function of 'haemoglobin' is to act as a carrier of oxygen from the lungs to all parts of the body.

HIV (human immuno-deficiency virus): range of illnesses caused by a retrovirus which seriously affects the body's immune system and thus its ability to protect itself. The virus is transmitted from one person to another by sexual contact and the direct passage of the virus via another material such as blood or an organ transplant.

Hospice: a specialist hospital that cares for people who are terminally ill and dying. The emphasis of treatment is on providing quality of life, including all appropriate methods of pain relief.

Huntington's Chorea: a hereditary disease characterised by involuntary movement and eventual dementia.

Isotopes: the collective name given to the four basic atomic elements: protons, neutrons, electrons and positrons. Certain radioactive isotopes (sometimes artificially produced) emit alpha, beta or gamma rays which are used in the diagnosis and treatment of cancer, as the rays can penetrate deeply into body tissue. Many substances present in the body can be targeted and tagged with radioactive material (label) to aid diagnosis. The radioactivity can be given in very small quantities and is easily identifiable by the rays it gives off, so its passage through the body can be detected. Gamma rays are used to treat deep-seated tumours.

Kaposi's sarcoma: malignant skin tumours originating from blood vessels and developing as a feature of AIDS (see above). The tumours form purple lumps starting at the feet and ankles and spreading to the hands and arms, respiratory tract and gut.

Lymph: the colourless, watery, fluid which circulates in the lymphatic system. It is similar to blood plasma (see below).

Lymphatic system: consists of capillaries (tread-like tubes), vessels, nodes (glands) and ducts and is similar to the blood system. The lymphatic system has two main functions: to help remove waste products from the cells and to play a major role in the body's defence system. As part of the nutritional mechanism of the body, individual cells are continually bathed in a tissue fluid which carries food, oxygen, water and waste products to and from the blood. The lymphatic system collects excess tissue fluid (lymph) containing waste products and transports it back to the blood stream, thus allowing a constant stream of fresh fluid to circulate around the cells. On its return journey the lymph fluid passes through nodes

255

which filter out bacteria and harmful substances. These nodes also produce new lymphocytes (white blood cells) which pass into the circulation, and antibodies and antitoxins to fight infection. Finally, the lymphatic vessels in the abdomen assist in the absorption of digested food, especially fat.

Lymphoid tissue: any tissue involved in the formation of lymph, lymphocytes and antibodies; for example, lymph nodes, certain glands, the spleen and the tonsils.

Lymphoma: a tumour of lymphoid tissue.

Malignant: a general term applied to diseases which are extremely serious. The word is mainly used to describe cancerous tumours that grow rapidly, invade healthy tissue and spread to distant organs. However, it is also applied to other conditions that occur in a form that is more serious than usual.

Metabolism: the term means 'tissue change' and includes all the processes (physical and chemical) that maintain the living body and produce energy to enable it to function.

Metastasis: the process by which malignant cancer spreads to other areas and organs of the body. The secondary sites are called metastases.

MRI (magnetic resonance imaging) scan: a type of whole body scan where the patient is placed within a magnetic field and the changes in the field are analysed. Special sensors measure the recovery time of the effects of the magnetic forces on tissues using the knowledge that different types of body tissues respond by giving off different signal times.

Oncologist: a specialist doctor involved in the treatment of cancer.

Oncology: the part of medicine (medical science) concerned with management and study of cancer.

Palliative care: treatment that is aimed at relieving symptoms and improving the quality of life, without bringing about a cure.

Plasma: the fluid part of the blood made up of serum (see below) and fibrinogen (the clotting material).

Platelets: a disk-shaped structure present in the blood involved in the clotting process.

Prognosis: a forecast of the predicted course and outcome of a disease given by a medically qualified practitioner, including an estimate of the person's remaining expectation of life.

Serum: the straw-coloured fluid which separates from blood cells, lymph and other material when clotting takes place.

'Staging' a cancer: a system that allows doctors to assess how a cancer is developing (with x-rays and scans) and to compare the cancer, with other cancers of the same type and at a similar stage. Most tumours are described using an internationally recognised set of features (criteria). For example, a diagnosis at 'stage 1' is earlier, and therefore better, than at 'stage 3'; numbers and letters are also used – 'T' stands for 'tumour', so T1 means a small growth whilst T4 equals a very large tumour; 'N' stands for 'nodes' and a number denotes the size of the involvement; 'M' indicates whether metastasis has taken place. Knowing the stage of a cancer enables the doctor to prescribe the most appropriate treatment and estimate the chances of recovery.

Ultrasound (ultrasonics): relates to sound frequencies above 15 kilocycles per second – well above the upper limits of the human ear. Ultrasound waves are used to examine the interior organs of the body (scan) and to treat soft tissue pain.

Urea and creatinine: are substances which are end products of protein metabolism and a constituents of urine.

Words ending in (suffix):
... ectomy: a suffix added to an organ name meaning removal of that organ ('ecto' means on the outside).
... itis: a suffix added to an organ name meaning a disease of that organ.
... oscopy: a suffix meaning internal examination of the body using a tube-shaped instrument called a '...scope', often with an integral light source. The procedure usually takes its name from the area of body to be investigated, for example, gastroscopy means examination of the stomach and the instrument used would be a gastroscope.

257

Useful addresses

Air Transport Users Council
CAA House
45–59 Kingsway
London WC2B 6TE
Tel: 020 7240 6061
Publishes a booklet Flight Plan, *which has a section for disabled passengers.*

Alzheimer's Society
Gordon House
10 Greencoat Place
London SW1P 1PH
Tel: 020 7306 0606
Care and research charity for people with all forms of dementia and their carers.

Alzheimer Scotland – Action on Dementia
22 Drumsheugh Gardens
Edinburgh EH3 7RN
Tel: 0131 243 1453
24-hour Freephone Dementia Helpline: 0808 808 3000
Provides specialist information and support for people with dementia and their carers in Scotland.

Aromatherapy Organisations Council
PO Box 19834
London SE25 6WF
Tel/Fax: 020 8251 7912 (10am–2pm)
For a list of qualified practitioners in your area.

Association of Reflexologists
27 Old Gloucester Street
London WC1N 3XX
Tel: 0870 567 3320
For a list of qualified practitioners in your area.

Bach Centre
Mount Vernon
Bakers Lane
Sotwell
Wallingford
Oxfordshire OX10 0PX
Tel: 01491 834678
For a list of trained practitioners and details of publications, tapes and educational material.

Breast Cancer Care
Klin House
210 New Kings Road
London SW6 4NZ
Freephone Helpline: 0808 800 6000
(10am–5pm weekdays, 10am–2pm Saturday)
Breast cancer information and support, prosthesis advice and counselling.

Bristol Cancer Help Centre
Grove House
Cornwallis Grove
Bristol BS8 4PG
Information Line: 0117 980 9500
Helpline: 0117 980 9505
Provides an holistic approach to complementary care for people with cancer.

British Association for Counselling and Psychotherapy (BACP)
1 Regent Place
Rugby
Warwickshire CV21 2PJ
Tel: 0870 4435252
Publishes a directory of counsellors in the UK.

British Colostomy Association
15 Station Road
Reading
Berkshire RG1 1LG
Tel: 0118 939 1537
Provides advice and support to patients and relatives.

British Complementary Medicine Association (BCMA)
PO Box 5122
Bournemouth BH8 0WG
Tel/Fax: 0845 345 5977
Publishes 'BCMA National Practitioner Register' listing practitioners who belong to member organisations.

British Herbal Medicine Association (BHMA)
Sun House
Church Street
Stroud
Gloucestershire GL5 1JL
Tel: 01453 751389
Provides an information service and list of qualified herbal practitioners.

British Holistic Medical Association (BHMA)
59 Lansdowne Place
Hove
East Sussex BN1 1FL
Tel: 01273 725951
For directory of members and book/tape list.

British Homeopathic Association (BHA)
15 Clerkenwell Close
London EC1R 0AA
Tel: 020 7566 7800
Provides an information service, newsletter, book list and names of homoeopathic practitioners.

British Nursing Association (BNA)
The Colonnades
Beaconsfield Close
Hatfield
Hertfordshire AL10 8YD
Tel: 01707 263544
Provides care assistants, home helps and qualified nurses to care for people in their own homes.

British Red Cross
9 Grosvenor Crescent
London SW1X 7EJ
Tel: 020 7235 5454 or look in the telephone directory for a local contact number.
For advice about arranging for equipment on loan.

CancerBACUP
3 Bath Place
Rivington Street
London EC2A 3JR
Tel: 020 7696 9003
Provides a range of services, support and publications for patients, relatives and professional workers.

Cancer Research UK
61 Lincoln's Inn Fields
London WC2A 3PX
Tel: 020 7242 0200
Promotes research into causes, symptoms and treatment and provides publications and information about cancer.

Care and Repair England
3rd Floor Bridgford House
Pavillion Road
West Bridgford
Nottingham NG2 5GJ
Tel: 0115 982 1527
Advice and practical assistance to older and disabled people and those on low incomes, to help them improve their home conditions.

Carers UK
20–25 Glasshouse Yard
London EC1A 4JT
Tel: 020 7490 8818
CarersLine: 0808 808 7777 (10am–12pm and 2pm–4pm, Monday to Friday)
Acts as the national voice of carers, raising awareness and providing support, information and advice.

Centre for Study of Complementary Medicine
51 Bedford Place
Southampton SO15 2DT
Tel: 0238 033 4752
For advice and details of specialist organisations.

Community Transport Association
Highbank
Halton Street
Hyde
Cheshire SK14 2NY
Tel: 0161 351 1475
Advice: 0161 367 8780
Services to benefit providers of transport for people with mobility problems. Also keeps a database of all Dial-a-Ride schemes.

Consumers Association
2 Marylebone Road
London NW1 4DF
Tel: 020 7770 7000
Publications on personal finance and law, including Wills and probate *and* What to do when someone dies.

Counsel and Care
Lower Ground Floor, Twyman House
16 Bonny Street
London NW1 9PG
Advice line: 0845 300 7585
(10am–1pm Monday–Friday)
*Offers free counselling, information and advice for older peo-
ple and carers, including specialist advice about using
independent agencies and the administration of trust funds
for one-off payments (for example, to cover the cost of respite
care).*

Crossroads – Caring for Carers
10 Regent Place
Rugby
Warwickshire CV21 2PN
Tel: 01788 573653
For respite care.

Cruse Bereavement Care
Cruse House
126 Sheen Road
Richmond
Surrey TW9 1UR
Tel: 020 8939 9530
Helpline: 0870 167 1677
*For all types of bereavement counselling and a wide range of
publications.*

C W Daniel Company Ltd
1 Church Path
Saffron Walden
Essex CB10 1JP
*For a booklist covering complementary therapies, including
Bach Flower Remedies.*

Dial-a-Ride
(see Community Transport Association)

Disability Benefits Centre
Warbreck House
Warbreck Hill
Blackpool FY2 0YE
Helpline: 08457 123 456
Information about exemption from road tax for vehicles used exclusively by or for disabled people.

Disabled Living Centres Council
Redbank House
4 St Chad's Street
Manchester M8 8QA
Tel: 0161 834 1044
For details of the Disabled Living Centre nearest you, where you can see aids and equipment.

Disabled Living Foundation
380–384 Harrow Road
London W9 2HU
Tel: 020 7289 6111
Helpline: 0845 130 9177
Information and advice about all aspects of daily living and aids and equipment for people with disability.

Disabled Persons Railcard Office
PO Box 1YT
Newcastle-upon-Tyne NE99 1YT
Helpline: 0191 269 0303
Minicom: 0191 269 0304
For railcard offering concessionary fares. An application form and booklet, Rail Travel for Disabled Passengers, *can be found at most larger stations or from the address above.*

Drinkline
85–89 Duke Street
Liverpool L1 5AP
Tel: 0800 917 8282
National alcohol helpline that provides confidential information, help and advice about drinking to anyone, including people worried about someone else's drinking.

Elderly Accommodation Counsel
3rd Floor
89 Albert Embankment
London SE1 7TP
Tel: 020 7820 1343
Computerised information about all forms of accommodation for older people (including nursing homes and hospices) and advice on top-up funding.

EXTEND
2 Place Farm
Wheathampstead
Hertfordshire AL4 8SB
Tel/Fax: 01582 832760
Provides exercise in the form of movement to music for people over 60 years, and less able people of all ages.

Federation of Independent Advice Centres
4 Dean's Court
St Paul's Churchyard
London EC4V 5AA
Tel: 020 7489 1800
Promotes the provision of independent advice services in the UK.

Health Development Agency
7th Floor, Holborn Gate
330 High Holborn
London WC1V 7BA
Tel: 020 7430 0850
Provides details of a wide range of leaflets and books promoting good health.

Help the Aged
207–221 Pentonville Road
London N1 9UZ
Tel: 020 7278 1114
Seniorline: 0808 800 6565
Advice and support for older people and their carers.

Helpbox
The Help for Health Trust
Freepost
Winchester SO22 5BR
Tel: 01962 849100
A computer database holding a comprehensive range of health-related information.

Holiday Care Service
2nd Floor, Imperial Buildings
Victoria Road
Horley
Surrey RH6 7PZ
Tel: 01293 774535
Textphone: 01293 776943
Information and advice on holidays, travel facilities and respite care for people with disabilities, on low income or with special needs.

Homeopathic Medical Association
6 Livingstone Road
Gravesend
Kent DA12 5DZ
Tel: 01474 560336
For a list of homoeopathic practitioners.

Hospice Information Service
St Christopher's Hospice
51–59 Lawrie Park Road
London SE26 6DZ
Tel: 020 8778 9252
For information about hospices and hospice care.

Ileostomy and Internal Pouch Support Group
Peverill House
1–5 Mill Road
Ballyclare BT39 9DR
Freephone: 0800 0184724
Help and support for people who have had their colon removed.

Independent Healthcare Association
Westminster Tower
3 Albert Embankment
London SE1 7SP
Tel: 020 7793 4620
For information about finding and paying for residential and nursing home care.

Independent Living (1993) Fund
PO Box 183
Nottingham NG8 3RD
Tel: 0115 942 8191
May fund very severely disabled people to buy in extra care if there is no one to fully meet their care needs.

Institute of Complementary Medicine (ICM)
PO Box 194
London SE16 7QZ
Tel: 020 7237 5165 (10am–3pm)
Advice and details of specialist organisations.

International Federation of Aromatherapists
182 Chiswick High Road
London W4 1PP
Tel: 020 8742 2605
For a booklist and details of qualified practitioners in your area.

International Federation of Professional Aromatherapists
82 Ashby Road
Hinckley
Leicestershire LE10 1SN
Tel: 01455 637987
For a booklist and details of qualified practitioners in your area.

International Stress Management Association UK
PO Box 348
Waltham Cross EN8 8ZL
Tel: 07000 780430
Publishes a wide range of materials to help reduce stress: leaflets, audio tapes, books and a newsletter.

Jewish Care
Stewart Young House
221 Golders Green Road
London NW11 9DQ
Tel: 020 8922 2000
Social care, personal support and residential homes for Jewish people.

Leukaemia Care Society
2 Shrubbery Avenue
Worcester WR1 1QH
Tel: 01905 330003
Freephone careline: 0800 169 6680
Provides information and financial assistance.

Lymphoma Association
PO Box 386
Aylesbury
Buckinghamshire HP20 2GA
Tel: 01296 619400
Provides an information and support service for patients and relatives.

Macmillan Cancerline
89 Albert Embankment
London SE1 7UQ
Tel: 020 7840 7840
Macmillan Cancerline: 0808 808 2020 (Monday–Friday, 9am–6pm)
Funds Macmillan nurses and works to improve the quality of life for cancer patients and their families through information, support and grant aid.

Marie Curie Cancer Care
89 Albert Embankment
London SE1 7TP
Tel: 020 7599 7777

(For Scotland)
29A Albany Street
Edinburgh EH1 3QN
Tel: 0131 456 3700
Provides inpatient centres and runs home nursing service for day and night care.

Motability
Goodman House
Station Approach
Harlow
Essex CM20 2ET
Customer Info Service: 01279 635666
Minicom: 01279 632273
Advice about cars, scooters and wheelchairs for disabled people.

National Association of Councils for Voluntary Service
Arundel Court
177 Arundel Street
Sheffield S1 2NU
Tel: 0114 278 6636
Promotes and supports the work of councils for voluntary service.

National Cancer Alliance
PO Box 579
Oxford OX4 1LB
Tel: 01865 793566
A voluntary group of patients and healthcare professionals formed to improve cancer services. Provides advice and information.

National College of Hypnosis and Psychotherapy
12 Cross Street
Nelson
Lancashire BB9 7EN
Tel: 01282 699378
Publishes an annual directory of practitioners.

National Federation of Spiritual Healers
Old Manor Farm Studio
Church Street
Sunbury on Thames
Middlesex TW16 6RG
Tel: 0845 123 2777
Advice and details of spiritual healers.

New World Music
16A Neal's Yard
Covent Garden
London WC2H 9DP
Tel: 020 7379 5972
For catalogue of relaxation music tapes.

Office of the Public Guardian
Hadrian House
Callander Business Park
Callander Road
Falkirk FK1 1XR
Tel: 01324 678300
Advice about powers of attorney in Scotland.

Public Guardianship Office
Archway Tower
2 Junction Road
London N19 5SZ
Tel: 0207 664 7327
Advice about powers of attorney in England and Wales.

Quitline
Tel: 0800 002 200
A freephone helpline that provides confidential and practical advice for people wanting to give up smoking.

RADAR (Royal Association for Disability and Rehabilitation)
12 City Forum
250 City Road
London EC1V 8AF
Tel: 020 7250 3222
Information about aids and mobility, holidays and leisure.

Research Institute for Consumer Affairs
30 Angel Gate
City Road
London EC1V 2PT
Tel: 020 7427 2460
Textphone: 020 7427 2469
Tests and evaluates goods and services for disabled and older people, including ordinary consumer products as well as special aids and equipment.

Royal College of Psychiatrists
17 Belgrave Square
London SW1X 8PG
Tel: 020 7235 2351
Publishes a range of information for dealing with anxieties, phobias, depression and bereavement.

St John Ambulance
Look in the telephone directory for local contact number.
For advice about arranging equipment on loan and first aid courses.

Samaritans
Tel: 08457 90 90 90 or see local telephone directory.

Society of Homeopaths
4A Artizan Road
Northampton NN1 4HU
Tel: 01604 621 400
For a list of homoeopathic practitioners.

SPOD (Association to Aid the Sexual and Personal Relationships of People with a Disability)
286 Camden Road
London N7 0BJ
Tel: 020 7607 8851
Telephone counselling: Monday and Wednesday 1.30–4.30pm; Tuesday and Thursday 10.30am–1.30pm.
Advice and information on sexual and personal relationships for people with a disability.

Sport England
16 Upper Woburn Place
London WC1H 0QP
Tel: 020 7273 1500
Provides general information about all sports.

Sue Ryder Care
Healthcare Office
PO Box 5044
Ashby de la Zouche
Leicestershire LE65 1ZP
Tel: 01332 694810
Provides specialist palliative care services at seven homes in the UK.

Tak Tent Cancer Support
Flat 5, 30 Shelley Court
Gartnavel Complex
Glasgow G12 0YN
Tel: 0141 211 0122
Provides an information and support group network across Scotland with drop-in resources centre at the above address.

Tenovus Cancer Information Centre
Velindre Hospital
Whitchurch
Cardiff CF14 2TL
Tel: 029 2019 6100
Provides a range of support services for people in Wales (in English and Welsh), with drop-in resources centre at the above address.

Tripscope
The Vassall Centre
Gill Avenue
Bristol BS16 2QQ
Helpline: 08457 585641
A travel and transport information service for older and disabled people in London and the southwest.

UK College of Complementary Health Care Studies
Wembley Centre for Health & Care
116 Chaplin Road
Wembley HA0 4UZ
Tel: 020 8795 6656/6178
For a list of qualified practitioners of therapeutic massage.

United Kingdom Home Care Association (UKHCA)
42B Banstead Road
Carshalton Beeches
Surrey SM5 3NW
Tel: 020 8288 1551
For information about organisations providing home care in your area.

University of the Third Age (U3A)
National Office
26 Harrison Street
London WC1H 8JG
Tel: 020 7837 8838
Day-time study and recreational classes. Send a sae for further information about classes for older people, or look in the telephone directory for local branch.

Volunteer Development England
New Oxford House
16 Waterloo Street
Birmingham B2 5UG
Tel: 0121 633 4555
*Information on matters related to volunteering, with a direc-
tory of volunteer bureaux and other publications.*

Winged Fellowship Trust
Angel House
20–32 Pentonville Road
London N1 9XD
Tel: 020 7833 2594
*Provides respite care and holidays for physically disabled
people, with or without a partner.*

About Age Concern

Caring for someone with cancer is one of a wide range of publications produced by Age Concern England, the National Council on Ageing. Age Concern works on behalf of all older people and believes later life should be fulfilling and enjoyable. For too many this is impossible. As the leading charitable movement in the UK concerned with ageing and older people, Age Concern finds effective ways to change that situation.

Where possible, we enable older people to solve problems themselves, providing as much or as little support as they need. A network of local Age Concerns, supported by many thousand volunteers, provides community-based services such as lunch clubs, day centres and home visiting.

Nationally, we take a lead role in campaigning, parliamentary work, policy analysis, research, specialist information and advice provision, and publishing. Innovative programmes promote healthier lifestyles and provide older people with opportunities to give the experience of a lifetime back to their communities.

Age Concern is dependent on donations, covenants and legacies.

Age Concern England
1268 London Road
London SW16 4ER
Tel: 020 8765 7200
Fax: 020 8765 7211

Age Concern Scotland
113 Rose Street
Edinburgh EH2 3DT
Tel: 0131 220 3345
Fax: 0131 220 2779

Age Concern Cymru
4th Floor
1 Cathedral Road
Cardiff CF11 9SD
Tel: 029 2037 1566
Fax: 029 2039 9562

Age Concern Northern Ireland
3 Lower Crescent
Belfast BT7 1NR
Tel: 028 9024 5729
Fax: 028 9023 5497

Other books in this series

The Carers Handbook series has been written for the families and friends of older people. It guides readers through key care situations and aims to help readers make informed, practical decisions. All the books in the series:

- are packed full of detailed advice and information;
- offer step-by-step guidance on the decisions which need to be taken;
- examine all the options available;
- are full of practical checklists and case studies;
- point you towards specialist help;
- guide you through the social services maze;
- are fully up to date with recent guidelines and issues;
- draw on Age Concern's wealth of experience.

Already published

Caring for someone with a sight problem
Marina Lewycka
£6.99   0–86242 381 3

Caring for someone with a hearing loss
Marina Lewycka
£6.99   0–86242–380-5

Caring for someone with arthritis
Jim Pollard
£6.99   0–86242–373-2

Caring for someone with diabetes
Marina Lewycka
£6.99   0–86242–374-0

Caring for someone with a heart problem
Toni Battison
£6.99   0–86242–371-6

Caring for someone with an alcohol problem
Mike Ward
£6.99   0–86242–372-4

Caring for someone who has had a stroke
Philip Coyne with Penny Mares
£6.99   0–86242–369-4

Caring for someone at a distance
Julie Spencer-Cingöz
£6.99   0–86242–367-8

Choices for the carer of an elderly relative
Marina Lewycka
£6.99   0–86242–375-9

Caring for someone who has dementia
Jane Brotchie
£6.99   0–86242–368-6

Caring for someone who is dying
Penny Mares
£6.99   0–86242–370-8

The Carer's Handbook: What to do and who to turn to
Marina Lewycka
£6.99   0–86242–366-X

Publications from Age Concern Books

Your Rights: A guide to money benefits for older people
Sally West

A highly acclaimed annual guide to the State benefits available to older people. It contains current information on Income Support, Housing Benefit and retirement pensions, among other matters, and provides advice on how to claim.

For more information, please contact Age Concern Books on 0870 44 22 044

Know Your Complementary Therapies
Eileen Inge Herzberg

People who practise natural medicine have many different ideas and philosophies, but they all share a common basic belief: that we can all heal ourselves – we just need a little help from time to time. Written in clear, jargon-free language, the book provides an introduction to complementary therapies, including acupuncture, herbal medicine, aromatherapy, homeopathy and osteopathy. Uniquely focusing on complementary therapies and older people, the book helps readers to decide which therapies are best suited to their needs, and where to go for help.

£9.99   0–86242–309–0

Staying Sane: Managing the stress of caring
Tanya Arroba and Lesley Bell

There is no doubt that providing care to people in their own homes can be very rewarding work – and at the same time very demanding.

The demands on the carer are many and can become overwhelming if not managed. The aim of this book is to increase the positive rewards associated with caring and demystify the topic of stress. In particular, this book will:

- increase awareness and understanding of stress;
- encourage awareness of the importance of dealing with stress as a carer;
- identify and explore the pressure and demands involved in caring;
- outline approaches for maintaining mental and emotional balance as a carer.

Complete with case studies and checklists, this is a book to help and support all carers in developing a clear strategy towards dealing positively with stress and staying sane.

£14.99   0–86242–267–1

If you would like to order any of these titles, please write to the address below, enclosing a cheque or money order for the appropriate amount (plus £1.99 p&p for one book; for additional books please add 75p per book up to a maximum of £7.50) made payable to Age Concern England. Credit card orders may be made on 0870 44 22 120. Books can also be ordered online at www.ageconcern.org.uk/shop

Age Concern Books
Units 5 and 6
Industrial Estate
Brecon
Powys LD3 8LA

We hope that this publication has been useful to you. If so, we would very much like to hear from you. Alternatively, if you feel that we could add or change anything, then please write and tell us, using the following Freepost Address: Age Concern, FREEPOST CN1794, LONDON SW16 4BR.

Bulk order discounts

Age Concern Books is pleased to offer a discount on orders totalling 50 or more copies of the same title. For details, please contact Age Concern Books on Tel: 0870 44 22 120.

Customised editions

Age Concern Books is pleased to offer a free 'customisation' service for anyone wishing to purchase 500 or more copies of the title. This gives you the option to have a unique front cover design featuring your organisation's logo and corporate colours, or adding your logo to the current cover design. You can also insert an additional four pages of text for a small additional fee. Existing clients include many of the biggest names in British industry, retailing and finance, the Trades Union Movement, educational establishments, the statutory and voluntary sectors, and welfare associations. For full details, please contact Sue Henning, Age Concern Books, Astral House, 1268 London Road, London SW16 4ER. Fax: 020 8765 7211. Email: hennins@ace.org.uk

Visit our Website at www.ageconcern.org.uk/shop

Age Concern Information Line/ Factsheets subscription

Age Concern produces 44 comprehensive factsheets designed to answer many of the questions older people (or those advising them) may have. Topics covered include money and benefits, health, community care, leisure and education, and housing. For up to five free factsheets, telephone: 0800 00 99 66 (7am–7pm, seven days a week, every day of the year). Alternatively you may prefer to write to Age Concern, FREEPOST (SWB 30375), ASHBURTON, Devon TQ13 7ZZ.

For professionals working with older people, the factsheets are available on an annual subscription service, which includes updates throughout the year. For further details and costs of the subscription, please write to Age Concern at the above Freepost address.

Index